Geriatric Oral Pathology

Second Edition

KMK Masthan MDS
Professor and Head
Department of Oral Pathology and Microbiology

S Raghavendra Jayesh MDS
Principal and Professor
Department of Prosthodontics

N Aravindha Babu MDS
Professor
Department of Oral Pathology and Microbiology

Sree Balaji Dental College and Hospital
Pallikaranai, Chennai, TN

CBS

CBS Publishers & Distributors Pvt Ltd

New Delhi • Bengaluru • Chennai • Kochi • Mumbai • Pune
Hyderabad • Kolkata • Nagpur • Patna • Vijayawada

Disclaimer

Science and technology are constantly changing fields. New research and experience broaden the scope of information and knowledge. The authors have tried their best in giving information available to them while preparing the material for this book. Although, all efforts have been made to ensure optimum accuracy of the material, yet it is quite possible some errors might have been left uncorrected. The publisher, the printer and the authors will not be held responsible for any inadvertent errors, omissions or inaccuracies.

Geriatric Oral Pathology
Second Edition

ISBN: 978-81-239-2299-7

Second Edition: 2014
First Edition: 2011

Published by Satish Kumar Jain for
CBS Publishers & Distributors Pvt Ltd
4819/XI Prahlad Street, 24 Ansari Road, Daryaganj, New Delhi 110 002, India.
Ph: 23289259, 23266861, 23266867 Website: www.cbspd.com
Fax: 011-23243014 e-mail: delhi@cbspd.com; cbspubs@airtelmail.in.
Corporate Office : 204 FIE, Industrial Area, Patparganj, Delhi 110 092
Ph: 4934 4934 Fax: 4934 4935 e-mail: publishing@cbspd.com; publicity@cbspd.com

Branches

- **Bengaluru:** Seema House 2975, 17th Cross, K.R. Road, Banasankari 2nd Stage, Bengaluru 560 070, Karnataka
  Ph: +91-80-26771678/79 Fax: +91-80-26771680 e-mail: bangalore@cbspd.com
- **Chennai:** 20, West Park Road, Shenoy Nagar, Chennai 600 030, Tamil Nadu
  Ph: +91-44-26260666, 26208620 Fax: +91-44-42032115 e-mail: chennai@cbspd.com
- **Kochi:** 36/14 Kalluvilakam, Lissie Hospital Road, Kochi 682 018, Kerala
  Ph: +91-484-4059061-65 Fax: +91-484-4059065 e-mail: kochi@cbspd.com
- **Mumbai:** 83-C, Dr E Moses Road, Worli, Mumbai-400018, Maharashtra
  Ph: +91-9833017933 e-mail: mumbai@cbspd.com
- **Pune:** Bhuruk Prestige, Sr. No. 52/12/2+1+3/2 Narhe, Haveli (Near Katraj-Dehu Road Bypass), Pune 411 041, Maharashtra
  Ph: +91-20-64704058, 64704059, 32392277 Fax: +91-20-24300160 e-mail: pune@cbspd.com

Representatives

- **Hyderabad** 0-9885175004
- **Nagpur** 0-9021734563
- **Vijayawada** 0-9000660880
- **Kolkata** 0-9831437309, 0-9051152362
- **Patna** 0-9334159340

Printed at : R P Printers, Noida

Foreword

PADMASHREE (Awardee)
Dr R SIVARAMAN
MS, DSc (Hony Causa) FICS, FAIS, FMMC, FABMS
Senior Surgeon, Geriatric Surgeon and G. Surgical Gastroenterologist

Pro Vice-Chancellor
Professor and Head
Geriatric Surgery
Senior Medical Supdt. (Admin).
Dean (Retd). Madrad Medical College and RI
Govt. General Hospital, Chennai - 03.
Governing Council and Senate Member
Chairman - Board of Studies for Higher Specialities
Member - Standing Academic Board
Member - Facutly of Surgery and Allied Specialities

Tamilnadu Dr. M.G.R. Medical University
Visiting Consultant, Apollo Hospitals
Chief Consultant Surgeon
T.N.E.B.H.Q. Hospital, Chennai - 2.
Guest Hospital : 7.00 to 9.00 p.m.
Ph : 2641 3420 Cell : 94440 82344
Expert Member
WHO Curriculum Development on Ageing
Hony. Panelist Geriatric Surgeon to
former President of India

A thorough knowledge of pathology both in medicine and dentistry is very essential for developing a good diagnostic skill. Diagnosis and treatment planning are the backbone of successful clinical practice. The advancement of dentistry and the quality of dental treatment are dependent upon the clinical application of basic sciences. Certainly no basic science could be more relevant to dentistry and dental specialty practice other than oral histology and pathology. Oral pathology is becoming widely recognized as an important area of formal study for dental graduates.

Geriatric dentistry is gaining a lot of importance these days and a very few books are available. This book is unique in the way that deals with oral pathology in geriatric patients. This books is unique in the way that deals with oral pathology, so it makes it very easy to understand. Another important feature of this book is that it deals with various systemic conditions which we come across in day-to-day practice and gives the management for these conditions too.

The sequential presentation of the subject form elementary principles of the more complicated systems in a simple and orderly manner will allow both the undergraduate students and practitioners to gain a better understanding of their application in clinical practice. It is a welcome sign that now books are forthcoming in our own country on these untouched aspects.

I am happy to compliment and congratulate Dr KMK Masthan and his coauthors for bringing out this well documented book for the benefit of dental students and practitioners.

Dr R Sivaraman

Preface

The focus of this book is the discussion of oral diseases and degenerative changes usually seen in the elderly population, i.e. above sixty years of age. Most of the diseases are not exclusive to old age but are more frequently observed in that age group.

Why this attempt to segregate regional pathology like oral pathology further into agewise distinctions? Geriatric medicine is the speciality that deals with the medical problems of the elderly and the professionals trained in that branch of medicine have shown and are showing exemplary acumen and results while treating senior citizens. What holds good in medicine must be applicable to dentistry also. Hence alongwith my coauthors I have decided to bring out a book on oral pathoses of the geriatric age group.

Literature as early as Charaka's bemoans the woes of old age and the diseases associated with old age. Some of the aches, complaints and diseases, are due to the wear and tear of the body. Oral cavity being a place which gets exposed to different types of food and trauma associated with speech processes develops diseases all the more easily in the old age. In addition, mouth acts as a mirror of the ailments of the other systems of the body which are numerous in the old age. Hence the oral diseases of the elderly merit an exclusive coverage like this book.

Most of the details and information given in this book are basically compilation of data from the standard textbooks of oral pathology and medicine, the names of which I have included under references. I owe the authors of those books my acknowledgment and thanks. I am grateful to my department staff, Dr Anita Nagarajan, postgraduate student, Dr Tathagata Bhattacharjee for doing the spadework in the compilation of data from different books and journals.

I and my coauthors have attempted to discuss the common oral pathoses of the elderly but this book is neither exhaustive nor comprehensive. Lapses, if any, are entirely my responsibility and the reader is most welcome to bring it to my notice at masthankmk@yahoo.com.

I think this book will serve its purpose if it helps the reader, be it a dentist or a medical practitioner or the care-giver to the elderly, to look for, understand and diagnose possible signs and symptoms or oral pathoses in the elderly.

KMK Masthan

Contents

Section I

1

Introduction

The World Health Organization's (WHO) definition of health as a state of complete physical, mental and social wellbeing. Ageing is a progressive, generalized impairment of function resulting in loss of adaptive response to stress and in increasing risk of agerelated diseases and disability. Ageing occurs at version levels: molecular, cellular, physiological, morphological, chronological, social, and behavioral.

Biological Changes in Ageing

Biological changes observed in ageing are an increase in chromosomal structural abnormalities, DNA crosslinking and frequency of single strand breaks, a decrease in DNA methylamine and loss of DNA telomeric sequences. The primary structure of protein is little affected while post-translational changes namely deamidation, oxidation, and crosslinking and non-enzymatic glycation increase significantly.

Ageing is more of a natural phenomenon mediated by genes and physiological changes.

Physiological Characteristics of Ageing

The major characteristic of the ageing is difference in physiologic process when the elderly is compared to the young adult. There is progressive constriction to the homeostatic reserve of every organ systema process termed 'homeostenosus', which starts in the 3rd decade of life. This process is gradual, independent of the organ system tends to vary from individual to individual and results from damage from intrinsic living process, damage caused by extrinsic factors and damage from age related diseases. Diet, environment, personal habit and genetic factors modify homeostenosis. This state of homeostasis is usually asymptomatic and has little impact on activities of daily living regardless of age.

Social Issues Related to Ageing and Health

Ageing is associated with several social problems, namely social isolation, proverty, apparent reduction in family support, inadequate housing, impairment of cognitic functioning, mental illness, windowhood, loss bereavement, limited options for living arrangement towards end of life. In addition, dependency due to physical or mental diseases is also an important issue involving human resource. All these problems have an impact on the quality of life in old age and health care at the time of need.

2

Tooth and Supporting Tissues

ENAMEL

PHYSICAL PROPERTIES

Enamel is a protective covering over the entire surface of crown and is hardest calcified tissue in the human body. Enamel withstands both shearing and impact forces well. An important property of enamel as it can undergo neither repair nor replacement. It is of variable thickness and attains maximum thickness of about 2 to 2.5 mm on the cusps and almost a knife edge at the cervical part of crown. The enamel was found to be thicker in the lingual surface of maxillary molars and in the buccal surfaces of mandible. These cusps are supporting cusps and increased enamel thickness over these surfaces are adaptation for functional demands. The structure and hardness of enamel render it brittle.

Fully formed enamel is most highly mineralized, consisting of approximately 96% inorganic and 4% organic material and water. Inorganic content of enamel is crystalline calcium phosphate (hydroxyapatite) and various ions strontium, magnesium, lead, and fluoride if present during enamel formation may be incorporated into the crystals. Enamel is semipermeable permitting complete or partial passage of certain molecules: C-labeled urea, iodine, etc. and dyes.

The color of enamel varies from light yellow to grayish white. Translucent enamel reflects yellow colour of dentin and teeth appears yellowish and grayish teeth having more opaque enamel. Enamel is a birefringent crystalline material, the crystals refracting light differently in different directions. Young enamel is white

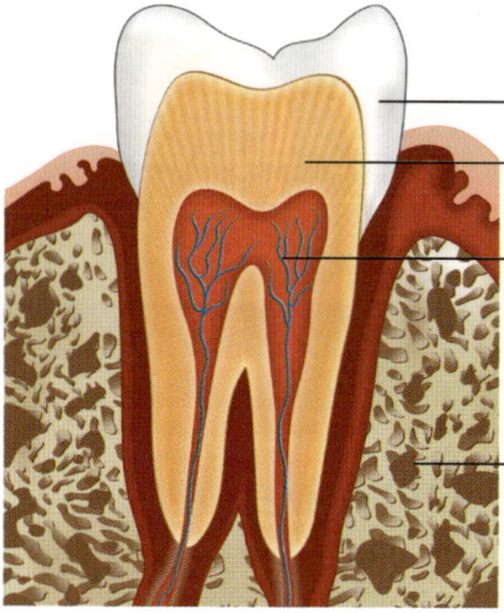

Fig. 2.1: Cross-section of a tooth

because, although light enters it readily, it is almost entirely internally reflected with no wavelengths differentially absorbed. This results in low translucency and the white color.

CHEMICAL PROPERTIES

The enamel consists of inorganic material (96%) and organic substance and water (4%)

Organic material consists of proteins. Two main groups of enamel proteins amelogenins and nonamelogenins. Amelogenins accounting 90% of enamel proteins and nonamelogenins constitute about 10% of enamel matrix proteins. Enamelin, ameloblastin and tuftelin are important proteins of this group. Inorganic material of the enamel is hydroxyapatite. The crystals of hydroxyapatite are arranged to form enamel rods or enamel prisms.

STRUCTURE OF ENAMEL

Rods

The enamel is composed of enamel rods or prisms, rod sheaths and in some regions a cementing interprismatic substance. The length of most rods is greater than the thickness of enamel because of the oblique rods and wavy course of rods. The rods located at the cusps are longer than those at cervical area. The enamel rods have clear crystalline appearance, permitting light to pass through them.

The rods are oriented at right angles to the dentin surface. In the incisal or tip of cusps they are almost vertical.

Incremental Lines of Retzius

It appears as brownish bands in ground sections of enamel. They illustrate the incremental pattern of the enamel, that is, the successive apposition of layers of enamel during formation of the crown. In longitudinal section they surround the tip of the dentin. In cervical parts of the crown they run obliquely. In transverse section they appear as concentric circles.

Enamel Lamellae

Enamel lamellae are thin, leaflike structures that extend from the enamel surface toward the dentinoenamel junction. They consists of organic material with little mineral content. Lamellae develop in planes of tension.

Enamel Tufts

Enamel tufts arise at dentinoenamel junction and reach into the enamel to about one-fifth to one-third of its thickness. An enamel tuft does not spring from a single area but is narrow, ribbonlike structure, the inner end of which arises at the dentin. Tufts consists of hypocalcified enamel rods and interprismatic substance. They extend in direction of the long axis of the crown. They are seen adundantly in horizontal and rarely in longitudinal sections.

Enamel Spindles

The odontoblastic processes pass across the dentinoenamel junction into the enamel. They are thickened at their end and hence termed as enamel spindles. They are hypomineralized or partially mineralized structures.

Age Changes in Enamel

Attrition: Enamel wears slowly with age, dependent on diet and masticatory habits. This is evidenced by a loss of vertical dimension of the crown and by flattening of the proximal contour.

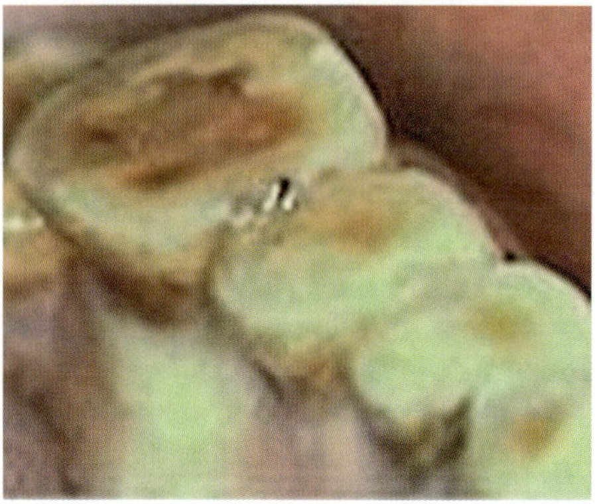

Fig. 2.2

Colour: Enamel darkens as age advances. Translucency of enamel increases with age and some of the colour of underlying dentin is then transmitted, resulting in a more yellow appearance. It seems to darken in colour, which may be in part due to reduced translucency of the tooth as secondary dentin forms and enamel thins and in part due to the accumulation of surface coatings and stains. The composition of the surface enamel alters as a result of additions and exchanges with the oral fluids. Fluorides can be beneficially be incorporated into surface enamel. This reduces its porosity and susceptibility to caries. Suggestive of aging change is greatly reduced permeability of older teeth to fluids. A decrease in permeability of enamel due to age is to increase in size of the crystal. An increase in size of crystal is due to ions acquired by it from the oral fluids.

Dental caries: Dental plaque is the primary source of micro-organisms (e.g. *Streptococcus mutans* and lactobacilli) causing coronal and root surface caries in elderly people. Individuals of all ages are susceptible to the development of dental plaque. However, following abstention from daily oral care, older individuals form plaque more rapidly than do younger people. Older people are more susceptible to new and recurrent tooth decay.

Treatment

Dental caries in elderly persons can be prevented by rigorous maintenance of oral hygiene, including brushing and flossing after

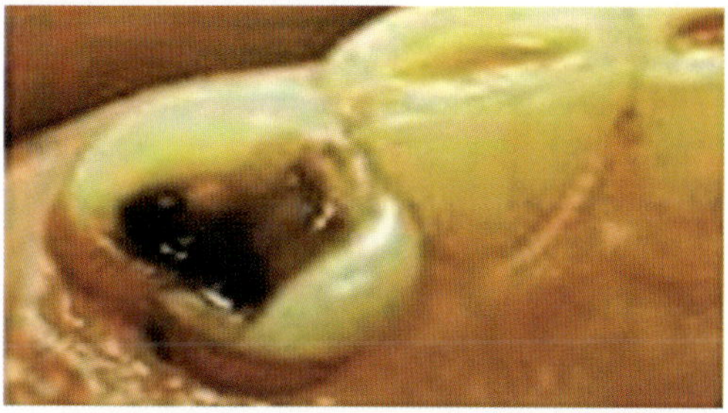

Fig. 2.3

each meal. The use of fluoride containing dentifrices and rinses can aid in remineralisation of existing decay and prevention of new carious lesions.

Early detection of caries can be restored with a variety of dental materials. In most circumstances, untreated caries will progress to severe or even total loss of tooth structure and possibly to pain, abscess formation, cellulitis and bacteremia. The enamel on attrition exposes dentin which results in sensitivity.

DENTIN

Dentin is mineralized tissue that forms the bulk of the tooth. In crown it is covered by enamel and in root by cementum. It is rigid but elastic tissue consisting of large number of dentinal tubules in collagen matrix. The dentinal tubules contain processes of odontoblast which are dentin forming cells. The distinguishing properties of dentin are it is sensitive and is formed throughout life.

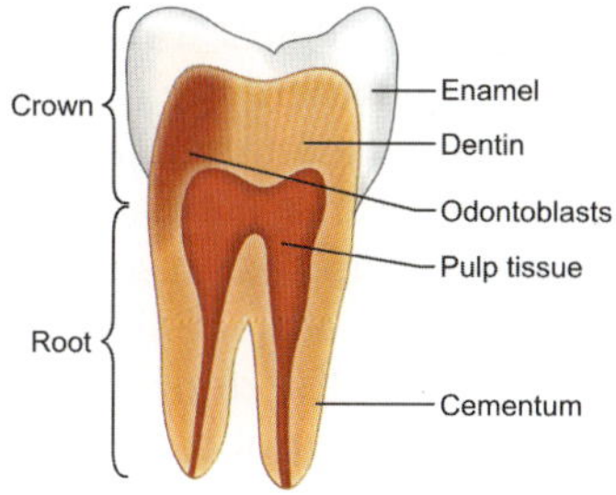

Fig. 2.4

PHYSICAL PROPERTIES

Dentin is pale yellow in colour and contributes to the appearance of the tooth through the translucent enamel. Dentin is harder than bone and cementum but softer than enamel. It has greater compressive, tensile and flexural strength than enamel due to tubular architecture and organic matrix. Dentin is permeable and it depends on the size and patency of the tubules.

CHEMICAL PROPERTIES

The gross composition of dentin approximates to 70% inorganic, 20% organic and 10% water by weight; 50% inorganic, 30% organic and 20% water by volume.

Organic matrix: Of dentin consists of fibrils embedded in an amorphous ground substance in which the crystallites are embedded. The principal collagen fibrils is the type I collagen. Traces of type III and type V collagen have also been detected.

Inorganic elements: The inorganic constituents of dentin consists of calcium, phosphorus, carbonate, sodium and magnesium.

STRUCTURE OF DENTIN

Dentinal Tubules

Dentinal tubules run from pulpal surface to dentinoenamel junction and cementoenamel junction. The dentinal tubules follow a curved, sigmoid course primary curvatures. The convexity of the primary curvatures nearest the pulp chamber faces rootward. In the root and beneath the cusps the dentinal tubules run in a straight course. The tubules are larger in diameter near pulp and lesser in diameter near dentinoenamel junction. The tubules are widely spaced near the dentinoenamel junction. The tubules also show changes in direction of much smaller amplitude. These are known as the secondary curvatures. In some region the secondary curvatures may coincide in adjacent tubules. This gives an appearance of a line crossing the dentin, a contour line of owen in low magnification. These are not commonly in dentin, but one such line is usually evident at the junction of primary and secondary dentin. Dentinal tubules branch. Many small branches appear to end blindly but some unite with branches of other tubules. Such branching of dentinal tubules is more profuse in the root dentin.

Peritubular Dentin

The walls of dentinal tubules of recently formed intertubular dentin at the pulp surface are comprised of mineralized type I collagen. With maturation, another type of dentin is deposited on the walls of the dentinal tubule, narrowing the size of lumen. This type of dentin is known as peritubular dentin (intratubular dentin), and deposition often eventually leads to obliteration of the tubule. Peritubular dentin differs from intertubular dentin in lacking collagenous fibrous matrix. Peritubular dentin is about 15% more mineralized than intertubular dentin. Peritubular dentin can be distinguished from intertubular dentin as a zone of increased radiographic and electron density.

Mantle Dentin

In the crown the first formed dentin is mantle dentin. It is slightly less mineralized than the rest of dentin. It varies in width from 20 to 150 microns. The collagen fibres are largely oriented perpendicular to the dentinoenamel junction.

Interglobular Dentin

Much of the mineral in dentin is deposited as globules or calcospherites. These in most areas, fuse to form a uniformly calcified tissue. However, in some areas especially beneath mantle dentin in crown and beneath the granular layer in root, the fusion is incomplete. When ground sections are viewed in transmitted light, internal reflection of the light makes the uncalcified, interglobular areas appear dark. Dentinal tubules pass without deviation through interglobular areas.

Granular Layer

In ground sections the periphery of the dentin in the root is marked by presence of a dark granular zone, the granular layer. The dentinal tubules in this area branch more profusely and loop back on themselves, creating air spaces in ground sections that result in internal reflection of transmitted light.

Circumpulpal Dentin

The circumpulpal dentin forms the bulk of dentin and is uniform in structure except at its edges where, peripherally, interglobular dentin marks incomplete initial mineralization and centrally, the mineralizing front represents ongoing mineralization.

Predenin

In demineralized sections stained with hematoxylin and eosin, the innermost layer of dentin, the predentin, has a distinct pale staining appearance. This reflects a difference in the composition of its matrix from that of the matrix of the mineralized circumpulpal dentin. The predentin is initially laid down dentin matrix before its mineralization.

AGE CHANGES IN DENTIN

Once the tooth is erupted and fully formed, dentin can undergo a number of changes that are either related to age or occur as a response to stimulus applied to the teeth, such as caries or attrition.

Secondary Dentin

The most conspicuous age associated change in dentin is the formation of secondary dentin. The primary and secondary dentin are delineated as a result of a change in direction of the dentinal tubules with coincidence of secondary curvature. This produces a particularly pronounced contour line of owen. The increased crowding of odontoblasts as secondary dentin formation continues throughout life, and the slower rate of deposition make the tubular pattern of secondary dentin a little less regular than somewhat closer together. Secondary dentin formation begins at the completion of root formation as the tooth comes into occlusion. Secondary dentin form rapidly in the pulpal floor. Its continuing deposition leads to smaller pulp chambers and narrower root canals in older patients.

Sclerotic Dentin

In physiological ageing, especially in root dentin, the tubules can become completely occluded with peritubular dentin to form translucent dentin. With age, translucent dentin is particularly

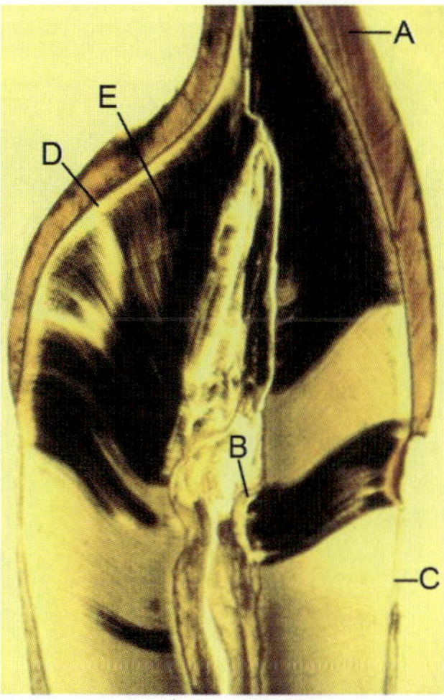

Fig. 2.5: (A) Enamel, (B) reparative dentin, (C) cementum, (D) mantle dentin, (E) circumpulpal dentin. Bend in tubules where primary and secondary dentin interface.

pronounced at the root apex and increases linearly with age. For this reason it is used in forensic dentistry to help determine the age of a person from the teeth.

The occluded dentinal tubules acquire same refractive index as the intertubular dentin. When a ground section of a root is placed in water (which has refractive index different from that of dentin), regions blocked by peritubular dentin will appear translucent, while regions with patent tubules will fill with water and appear opaque. The dentinal tubules become infilled at the root apex adjacent to the cementum and extend cervically and towards the root canal with age. In cross-section, translucent zones have a butterfly shape owing to the convergence of the tubules pulpally, being wider at the mesial and distal margins.

Tertiary Dentin

The dental pulp may be induced to produce calcified material in addition to its usual primary and secondary dentin by a variety of outside stimuli including caries, attrition, cavity preparation, microleakage around restorations and trauma. Stimuli of different types and extent may be applied to teeth at different stages of

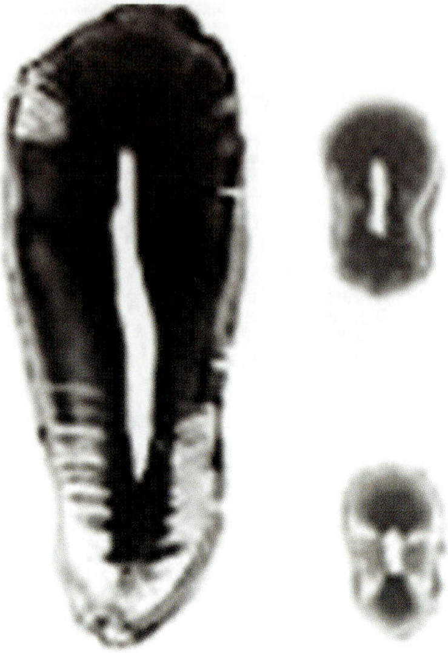

Fig. 2.6

development or ageing, resulting in a response tissue that may vary considerably in appearance and composition—it may resemble secondary dentin in having regular tubular structure; it may have a few and/or irregularly arranged tubules; or it may be relatively atubular. The continuity of dentinal tubules between normal dentin and tertiary dentin will therefore be lost in many instances. Wide range of above said presentations has given it variety of names, including irregular secondary dentin, reparative dentin, reactionary dentin, response dentin and osteodentin.

Dead Tracts

If the primary odontoblasts are killed by an external stimulus, or retract before peritubular dentin occludes the tubules, empty tubules will be left. They may be sealed at the pulp ends by tertiary dentin. When ground sections are prepared the mounting medium will not enter these sealed off tubules and they remain air filled. Under transmitted light they appear dark. This appearance, which is partly due to pulpal response and partly due to preparatory procedure, has been termed a dead tracts.

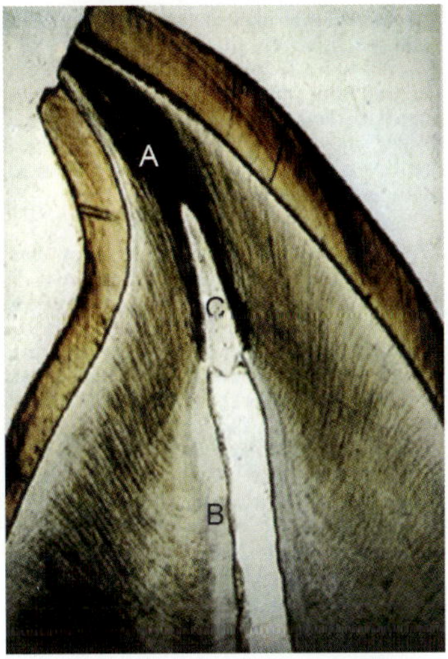

Fig. 2.7: (A) Dead tracts, (B) secondary dentin, (C) reparative dentin

Treatment

The treatment of destroyed tooth morphology and exposed dentin due to dental caries, attrition, abrasion, and erosion is dent-inbonding techniques. Attrition of enamel with mild exposure of dentin can be managed by desensitizing pastes. Severe attrition of enamel with large exposure of dentin can be treated by performing intentional root canal treatment and crown placement.

PULP

Dental pulp consists of soft connective tissue and occupies the centre of each tooth. Pulp is housed in the pulp chamber of the crown and in the root canal of the root. The pulp present in the crown is called coronal pulp and pulp present in the root is called radicular pulp.

The total volumes of all the permanent teeth pulp is 0.38 cc and the mean volume of a single adult human pulp is 0.02 cc.

CORONAL PULP

Coronal pulp in young individuals resembles the shape of outer surface of the crown dentin. Coronal pulp has six surfaces: The

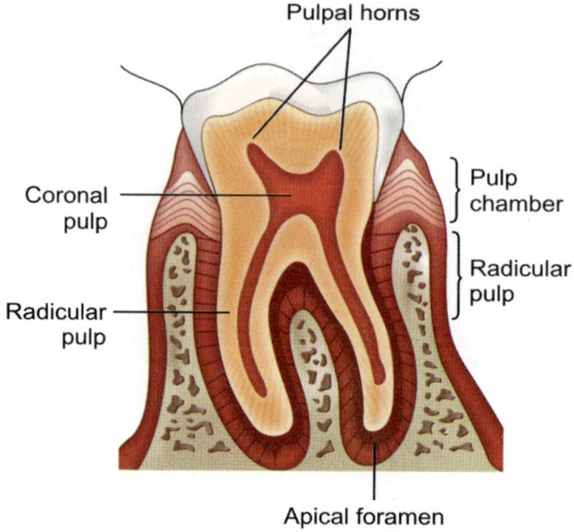

Fig. 2.8: Pulpal horns

roof or occlusal, the mesial, the distal, the buccal, the lingual and the floor. The protrusions of the pulp into the cusps of each crown are the pulp horns. The number of these horns thus depends on the cuspal number. The cervical region of the pulp organs constricts as does the contour of the crown, and at this zone the coronal pulp joins the radicular pulp.

Age Change

Continuous deposition of dentin causes the pulp to become small with age. This is not uniform through coronal pulp but progresses faster on the floor than on the roof or side walls.

RADICULAR PULP

Radicular or root pulp is that pulp extending from the cervical region of the crown to the root apex. In anterior teeth the radicular pulps are single and posterior ones multiple. They are not always straight and vary in size, shape and number. The radicular portions of the pulp are continuous with the periapical connective tissues through the apical foramen or foramina. The dentinal walls taper, and the shape of the radicular pulp is tubular. During root formation the apical root end is a wide opening limited by an epithelial diaphragm. As growth proceeds, more dentin is formed, so that when the root of the tooth has matured the radicular pulp is narrower. The apical pulp canal becomes smaller also because of apical cementum deposition.

Apical Foramen

Maxillary teeth in adult: Apical foramen - 0.4 mm

Mandibular teeth slightly smaller - 0.3 mm

Changes in the Location and Shape of the Apical Foramen

A tooth may be tipped from horizontal pressure, or it may migrate mesially, causing the apex to tilt in the opposite direction. Under these conditions the tissues entering the pulp through the apical foramen may exert pressure on the one wall of the foramen, causing resorption. At the same time, cementum is laid down on the opposite side of the apical root canal, resulting in a relocation of the original foramen.

Accessary Canals

Accessary canals leading from radicular pulp to the periodontal tissue occur anywhere laterally along the root but are numerous in the apical third of the root.

They are clinically significant in spread of infection, either from the pulp to the periodontal ligament or vice versa.

Histology of the Pulp

Central region of both the coronal and the radicular pulp contains large nerve trunks and blood vessels.

Peripherally the pulp is circumscribed by the specialized odontogenic region composed of

- Odontoblastic zone
- Cell-free zone (Weil's zone)
- Cell-rich zone

Odontoblastic Zone

Odontoblasts are second most prominent cell in the pulp. They reside adjacent to the predentin with cell bodies in the pulp and cell processes in the dentinal tubules. The cell bodies of the odontoblasts are columnar with large oval nuclei which fill the basal part of the cell. An active odontoblast is elongated whereas a resting cell is stubby. The active cell has basally placed nucleus and a basophilic cytoplasm. The resting cell has little cytoplasm but a more *hematoxyphilic nucleus*. The form and arrangement of the bodies of the odontoblasts are not uniform throughout the pulp. They are more cylindrical and longer (tall columnar) in the crown and more cuboidal in the middle of the root. Close to the apex of an adult tooth the odontoblasts are ovoid and spindle shaped.

Cell-free Zone

The cell-free zone is a space in which the odontoblast may more pulp ward during tooth development and to limited extent in functioning teeth.

Cell-rich Zone

It is composed principally of fibroblasts and undifferentiated mesenchymal cells.

Fibroblasts

Fibroblasts are most numerous cell type in the pulp. They function in collagen fiber formation throughout the pulp during the life of the tooth. They have the typical stellate shape and extensive processes that contact and are joined by intercellular junctions to the processes of other fibroblasts.

Age Change in Fibroblast

In older pulp they appear rounded or spindle shaped with short processes and exhibit fewer intracellular organelles. They are then termed fibrocytes.

Undifferentiated Mesenchymal Cells

They are primary cells in the very young pulp, but a few are seen in the pulps after root completion. They are polyhedral in shape with peripheral processes and large oval staining nuclei and appear larger than fibroblasts. They are found along pulp vessels, in the cell rich zone and scattered throughout the central pulp.

Intercellular Substances

The intercellular substance is dense and gel like in nature, varies in appearance from finely granular to fibrillar and appears more dense in some areas, with clear spaces left between various aggregates. It is composed of both acid mucopolysaccharides and protein polysaccharide compounds (glycosaminoglycans and proteoglycans)

Regressive or Age Change in Pulp

Cellular Changes

Cells are characterized by a decrease in size and number of organelles. Typical active pulpal fibroblast has abundant rough endoplasmic reticulum notable golgi complex and numerous mitochondria with well developed cisternae.

The fibroblasts in aging pulp exhibit less perinuclear cytoplasm and possessing, thin cytoplasmic processes. The intracellular organelles are reduced in number and size, e.g. mitochondria and endoplasmic reticulum.

Vascular Changes

Atherosclerotic plaques may appear in pulpal vessels. The outer diameter of vessel walls becomes greater as collagen fibers increase in the medial and advential layers. Calcifications are found that surrounded vessels, unusually found most often in the region near the apical foramen. The capillary endothelium shows numerous pinocytotic vesicles, microvesicles and microfilaments in the elderly lipid like vacuoles, glycogen granules and many golgi complexes are present. With age blood flow decreases.

Fibrosis

In the aging pulp accumulations of both diffuse and fibrillar components as well as bundles of collagen fibers usually appear. Fiber bundles are arranged in longitudinal bundles in the radicular pulp and in more random more diffuse arrangement in the coronal area. The increase in fibers in the pulp organ is gradual and is generalized throughout the organ. External trauma such as dental caries and deep restorations usually causes a localized fibrosis and scarring effect. Collagen increase is noted in the medial and adventitial layers of blood vessels as well. The increase in collagen fibers may be more apparent than actual, being attributable to the decrease in the size of the pulp, which makes the fibers present occupy less space and hence they become more concentrated without increasing in total volume.

Size of Pulp Space

The continual dentin deposition results in decreasing volume of pulp chamber and root canal. In older teeth the root canal is often no more than a thin channels; indeed the root canal can on occasion appear to be obliterated almost completely.

Sensitivity of Pulp

With age come a loss and a degeneration of myelinated and unmyelinated axons that correlate with an age related reduction in sensitivity.

Pulp Stones/Denticles

Pulp stones are nodular, calcified masses appearing in either or both the coronal and root portions of the pulp organ. They are usually asymptomatic unless they impinge on nerve or blood vessels. They have been seen in functional as well as embedded unerupted teeth.

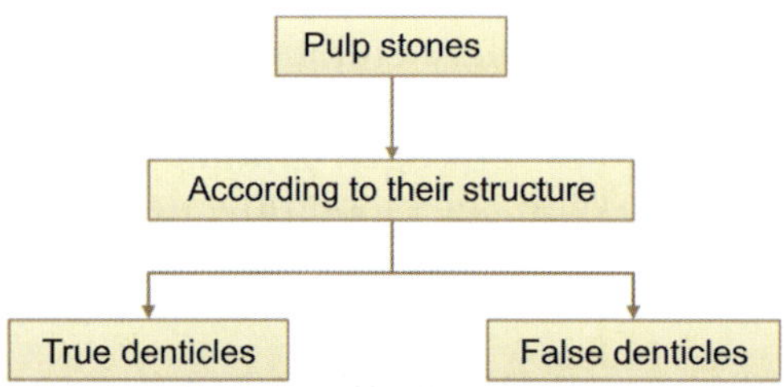

True denticles are similar in structure to dentin in that they have dentinal tubules and contain the process of odontoblasts that formed them and that exist on their surface. True denticles are rare and located close to the apical foramen. A theory has been advanced that the development of true denticle is caused by inclusion of remnants of epithelial remnants induce the cells of the pulp to differentiate into odontoblasts, which then forms the dentin.

False denticles do not exhibit dentinal tubular pattern but appear as concentric layers of calcified tissue. Calcification occurs:

- Within a bundle of collagen fibers
- Appear in a location in pulp free of collagen accumulations
- Some false pulp stones arise around blood vessels

Calcification of thrombi in blood vessels called phleboliths, may also serve as nidi for false denticles. All denticles begin as small nodules but increase in size by incremental growth on their surface.

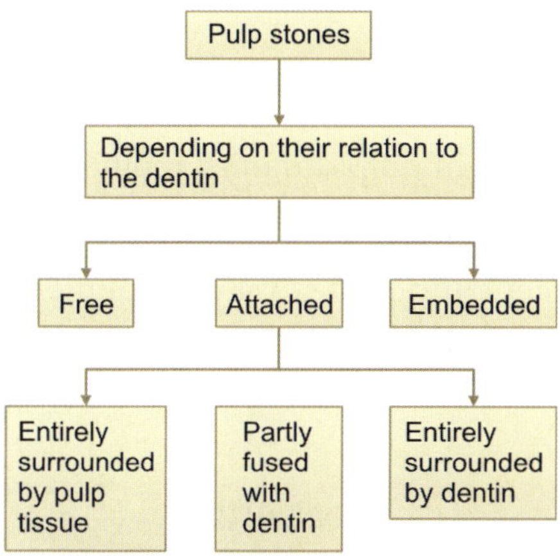

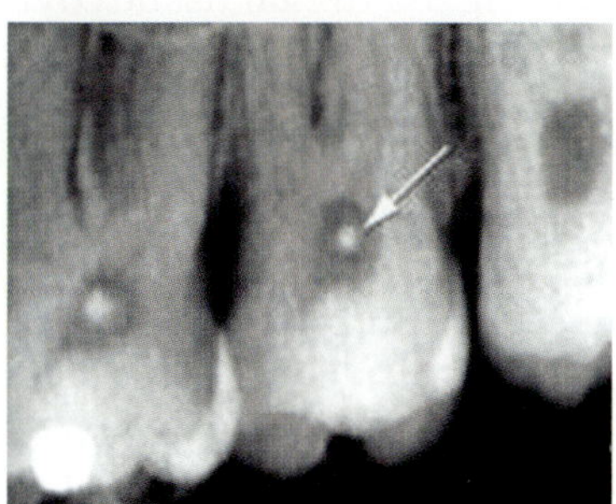

Fig. 2.9

The incidence and size of pulp stones increases with age. Denticles are more frequently seen in coronal pulp.

A statistically significant relationship has been found between patients with cardiovascular disease and presence of pulp stones. This finding suggests the usefulness of dental radiographs to identify patients with cardiovascular diseases for further screening and evaluation.

Diffuse Calcifications

Diffuse calcifications appear as irregular calcific deposits in the pulp tissue, usually following collagenous fiber bundles or blood vessels. They develop into larger masses but usually persists as fine calcified spicules. Diffuse calcifications are usually found in the root canal. These calcifications may be classified as dystrophic calcification.

Treatment

Age related changes in pulp diminish tooth sensitivity and pain perception, reduce responsiveness to pulp testing and usually decrease the need for local anaesthesia for dental procedures. Presence of larger pulp stones may encounter problem while performing root canal treatment, hence any restriction for instrumentation during root canal treating should be checked for pulp stones.

CEMENTUM

Cementum is the mineralized dental tissue covering the anatomic roots of human teeth. It begins at the cervical portion of the tooth at the cementoenamel junction and continues to the apex. Cementum furnishes a medium for attachment of collagen fibers that bind the tooth to surrounding structures. Cementum shares some physical, chemical and structural characteristics of compact bone; however cementum is avascular and non-innervated unlike bone.

Cementum is thinnest at the cementoenamel junction (20–50 μm) and thickest toward the apex (150–200 μm). Apical foramen is surrounded by cementum.

Physical Characteristics

The hardness of fully mineralized cementum is less than that of dentin. Cementum is light yellow in color and can be distinguished from enamel by its lack of luster and its darker hue.

Chemical Composition

Inorganic substances – 45 to 50%
Organic material and water – 50 to 55%

Inorganic portion mainly consists of calcium and phosphate in the form of hydroxyapatite. Numerous trace elements are found in cementum in varying amounts. Organic portion of cementum consists primarily of type I collagen and protein polysaccharides (proteoglycans). The other types of collagen seen are type III, V, VI and XII.

The non-collagenous protein plays important roles in matrix deposition, initiation and control of mineralization and matrix remodeling. Many non-collagenous proteins are common to both cementum and bone. Bone sialoprotein and osteopontin are two such major proteins that fill up the large interfibrillar spaces.

Structure of Cementum

Light microscopic observation reveal two basic types of cementum. They are usually classified on the basis of presence of cementocytes (cellular cementum) or its absence (acellular cementum). It can also be classified on the basis of the type of fibers (intrinsic/extrinsic fibers) presence or their absence (afibrillar cementum). Thus by combining the types of fibers-extrinsic and intrinsic fibers and the presence or absence of cementocytes, different types of cementum are described. Acellular extrinsic fiber cementum, cellular intrinsic fiber cementum and acellular afibrillar cementum are usually described.

Cementoenamel Junction

The relation between cementum and enamel at the cervical region of teeth is variable. In approximately 30% of all teeth, cementum meets the cervical end of enamel in a sharp line. In about 10% of all the teeth, enamel and cementum do not meet. In approximately

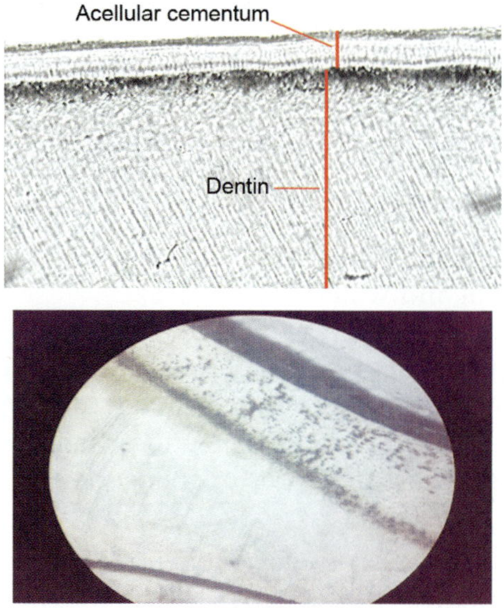

Fig. 2.10: Cellular cementum

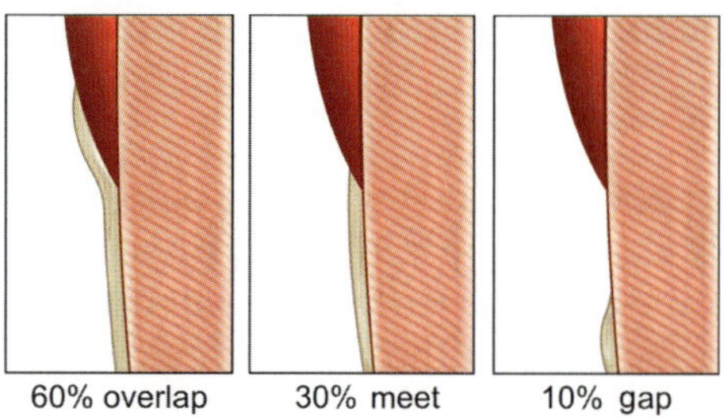

Fig. 2.11: Cementoenamel junction

60% of the teeth, cementum overlaps the cervical end of enamel for a short distance.

Cementodentinal Junction

The dentin surface upon which cementum is deposited is relatively smooth in permanent teeth. The cemental fibers intermingle with the dentinal fibers at the cementodentinal junction more in cellular cementum than in acellular cementum and aids in attachment of cementum to the dentin. Since collagen

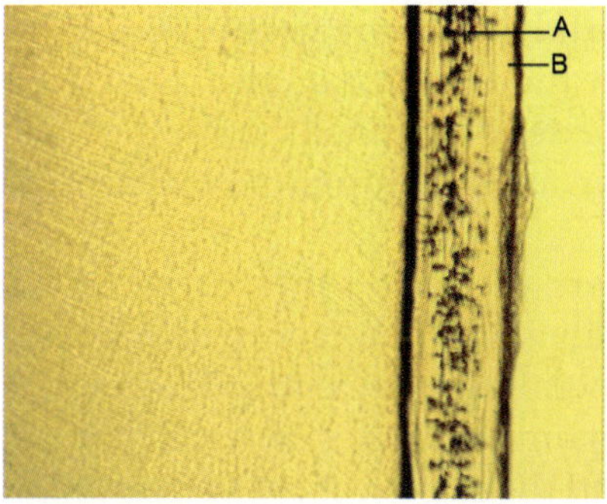

Fig. 2.12: Cementodental junction: (A) Cementocytes, and (B) cellular cementum

fibrils of cementum and dentin intertwine at their interface in a complex fashion, it is not possible to precisely determine which fibrils are of dentinal and which are of cemental origin.

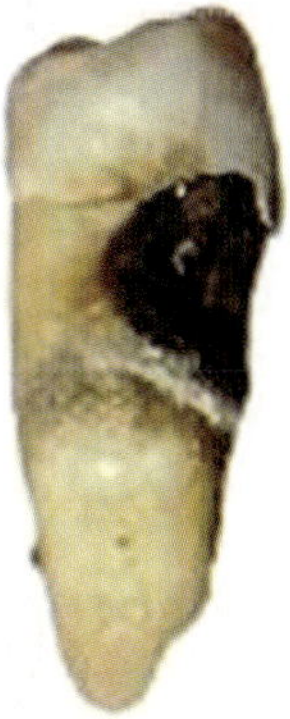

Fig. 2.13

Age Changes in Cementum

Prominent age changes seen in cementum is scalloping. Cementum thickness is reduced with age. Recession of gingiva in older persons exposes cementum and root caries is commonly encountered. These lesions appears as well defined and discoloured defects on cementum or at cementoenamel junction

Treatment

The treatment of root caries is by restorative procedures.

PERIODONTAL LIGAMENT

The periodontium is connective tissue organ covered by epithelium and attaches the teeth to the bones of the jaws and provides a continually adapting apparatus for support of the teeth during function. Periodontium comprises of cementum, periodontal ligament, bone lining the tooth socket and the part of gingiva facing the tooth.

The periodontal ligament occupies the periodontal space, located between the cementum and periodontal surface of the alveolar bone. It extends coronally to the most apical part of lamina propria of gingiva and is continuous with dental pulp at the apical foramen.

Collagen fibers of periodontal ligament are embedded in cementum and alveolar bone and provide soft-tissue continuity between the mineralized connective tissues of the periodontium.

Periodontal ligament ranges in width from 0.15 to 0.38 mm. It is thinnest around the middle third of the root, with an hour glass appearance.

Age change in thickness: Periodontal ligament shows progressive decrease in thickness with age

Young adult – 0.21 mm
Mature adult – 0.18 mm
Older adult – 0.15 mm

Periodontal ligament space appears to be 0.4 to 1.5 mm in radiographs. It is seen as radiolucency area between the radiopaque lamina dura of the alveolar bone proper and radiopaque cementum. The periodontal ligament space of permanent teeth is narrower than that of the deciduous teeth.

Structures of Periodontal Ligament

Periodontal ligament is a fibrous connective tissue and is cellular and contains numerous blood vessels. It comprises extracellular matrix consisting of fibers and ground substances

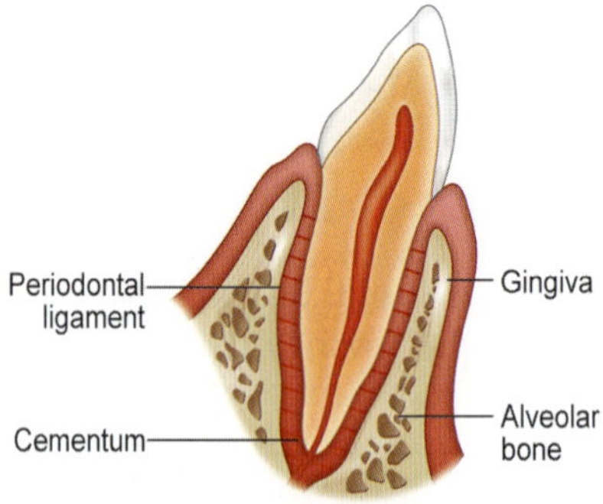

Fig. 2.14

- Fibers of periodontal ligament: Collagen fibers
- Matrix of periodontal ligament: Proteins and polysaccharides

Principal Fibers of Periodontal Ligament

- *Alveolar crest fiber bundle group:* From the alveolar crest of alveolar bone to the cervical cementum
- *Oblique fiber bundles:* In the middle third of the root
- *Horizontal group:* Coronal third of the root
- *Apical fiber group:* Apical root

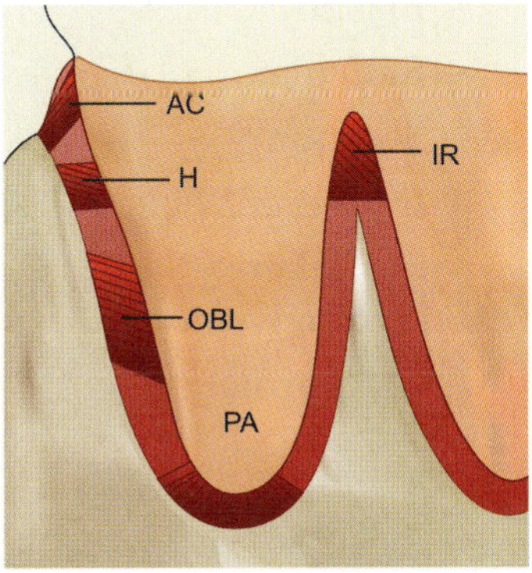

Fig. 2.15: AC—Alveolar crest fibers; H—Horizontal; OBL—Oblique fibers PA—Apical fibers; IR—Inter-radicular fibers

- *Inter-radicular group:* In the inter-radicular part of multirooted teeth

Cells of Periodontal Ligament

The principal cells of the healthy, functioning periodontal ligament are concerned with the synthesis and resorption of alveolar bone and fibrous connective tissue of the ligament and cementum.

1. Synthetic cells – Fibroblasts
   – Osteoblasts
   – Cementoblasts

2. Resorptive cells – Osteoclasts
   – Fibroblasts
   – Cementoclasts
3. Progenitor cells
4. Epithelial rests of Malassez
5. Defense cells – Mast cells
   – Macrophages
   – Eosinophils

Extracellular substances of Periodontal Ligament

Fibers – Collagen
– Elastic
– Reticular
– Secondary
– Indifferent fiber plexus
– Oxytalan

Ground substance – Proteoglycans
– Glycoproteins

Structures Present in Connective Tissue

- Blood vessels
- Lymphatics
- Nerves
- Cementicles

Cementicles

Cementicles are calcified bodies sometimes found in the periodontal ligament. These bodies are seen in older individuals and they may remain free in the connective tissue. They may fuse into large calcified masses or they may be joined with the cementum.

As cementum thickens with advancing age, it may envelop these bodies. When they are adherent to the cementum, they form excementoses. Origin of these calcified bodies is not established. It is possible that degenerated epithelial cells form the nidus for their calcification.

Age Changes

Periodontal ligament: The cell number and cell activity decreases with aging. Age change leading to scalloping of bone and cementum, and the periodontal ligament attaches to the peaks of these scallops than over the entire surface as seen in younger periodontium. This remarkable change affects the supporting structures of the teeth.

With aging the activity of PDL tissue decreases because restricted diets and therefore normal functional stimulation of the tissue is diminished. Any loss of gingival height related to gingival and periodontal disease promotes destructive changes in the periodontal ligament. The periodontal ligament width starts to dwindle in non-functional teeth.

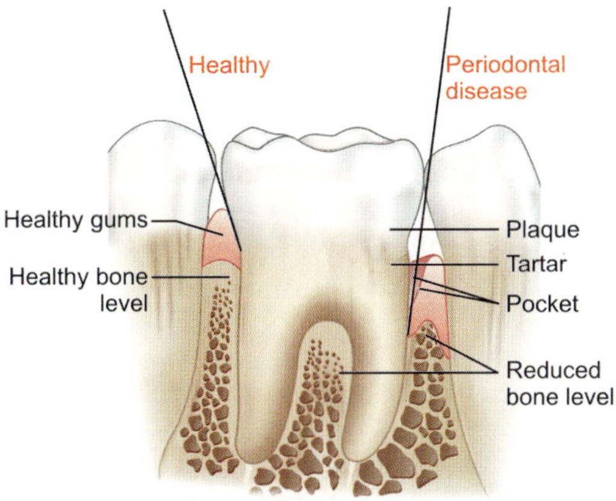

Fig. 2.16

Age related immunologic changes and histologic changes in periodontal tissues could alter the host response to dental plaque microorganisms, affecting the patient's ability to respond to periodontal treatment.

Treatment

Treatment of periodontal diseases in elderly patient requires an assessment of patient's attitude and expectations, previous dental or periodontal treatments, current oral health status, oral hygiene practices, medical conditions, medications. For most elderly patients, a non-surgical approach with scaling and root planning and meticulous daily oral hygiene is indicated. Gingival recession, furcation involvement and large embrasure spaces make periodontal treatment and maintenance more difficult in older patients. Advanced age is not a contraindication for periodontal surgery although certain systemic conditions (e.g. congestive heart failure, diabetes) and medications (e.g. corticosteroids, anti-coagulants) may complicate surgical procedures. If periodontal disease is believed to arise from patient's medical conditions and their treatment, then a systemic approach to oral health management is required.

BONE

Bone is a living tissue, which makes up the body skeleton and is one of the hardest structures of the animal body. Bone possesses a certain degree of toughness and elasticity. It provides shape and support for the body. It provides site of attachment for tendons and muscles, which are essential for locomotion. It protects vital organs of the body. Bone serves as a storage site for minerals and provides the medium, marrow for development and storage of blood cells.

Composition of Bone

Bone is connective tissue composed of cells, fibers and ground substance. The intercellular substance of bone consists of organic and inorganic substances. The inorganic part of bone is made of bone minerals.

Mineral component: Hydroxyapatite crystals, carbonate content and low ratio than the pure hydroxyapatite.

Bone crystals are in the form of thin plates or leaflike structures.

Organic matrix: Collagen and non-collagenous.

All bones have a dense outer sheet of compact bone and a central medullary cavity. The cavity is filled with red or yellow bone marrow in living bone. This cavity show a network of bone trabeculae.

Compact bone is surrounded by condensed fibrocollagen layer, the periosteum.

The inner surfaces of compact and cancellous bone are covered by a thin cellular layer called endosteum.

Bone Cells

Osteoblasts: These are mononucleated cells responsible for the synthesis and secretion of the macromolecular organic constituents of bone matrix. It is derived from osteoprogenitor cells of mesenchymal origin, which are present in the bone marrow and other connective tissues periosteum also serves as an important reservoir of osteoblasts, particularly during childhood growth, after skeleton fractures or with bone forming tumors.

Osteocytes: As the osteoblasts from the bone matrix, they get entrapped within the matrix they secrete and are called osteocytes. The number of osteoblasts that become osteocytes depends on the rapidity of bone formation.

Osteoclast: It is a type of bone cell that removes bone tissue by removing the mineralized matrix of bone.

Bone remodeling: bone is a highly dynamic connective tissue with a capacity for continuous remodeling. The two principal cell types osteoclast and osteoblast are the major effectors in the turnover of bone matrix. At any given time, the process of bone synthesis and bone breakdown go on the simultaneously and the status of the bone represents the net result of a balance between the two process. This phenomenon is called *coupling* of bone resorption and formation.

The main functions of remodeling are to present accumulation of damaged and fatigued bone by regeneration of new bone, allow the bone to respond to changes in mechanical forces and to facilitate mineral homeostasis.

Bone turnover rates of 30 to 100 % per year are common in rapidly growing children. The osteoclasts tunnel into surface of bone, which lasts for three weeks. Osteoclasts travel along the blood vessels, resorb the bone forming resorption tunnel. After sometime resorption ceases and osteoclasts are replaced by osteoblasts. These osteoblasts lay down new bone, encircling a vessel.

Alveolar bone: The alveolar process bone may be defined as that part of the maxilla and mandible that forms and supports the sockets of the teeth. As a result of its adaptation to function, two parts of the alveolar process can be distinguished. The first consists of a thin lamella of bone that surrounds the root of the tooth and gives attachment to principal fibers of periodontal ligament. This is alveolar bone proper. The second part is the bone that surrounds the alveolar bone proper and gives supports to the socket this has been called supporting alveolar bone.

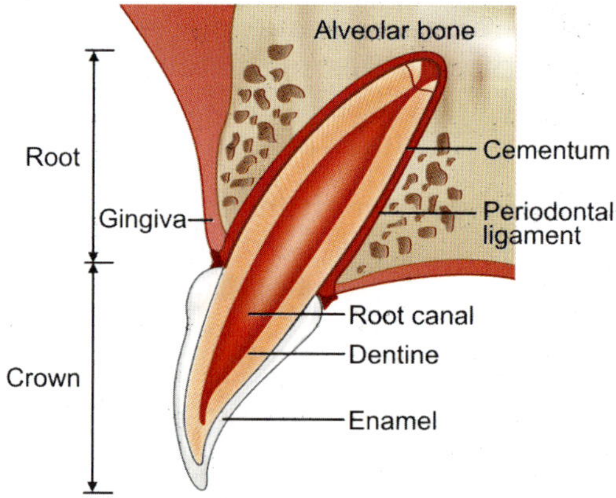

Fig. 2.17

Alveolar bone proper: The alveolar bone proper consists partly of lamellated and partly of bundle bone.

Lamellated bone: Some lamellae of the lamellated bone are arranged roughly parallel to the surface of the adjacent marrow spaces, whereas others form haversian systems.

Bundle bone: Bundle bone is that bone in which the principal fibers of periodontal ligament are anchored, radiographically it is also referred to as the lamina dura, because of increased radiopacity.

The supporting alveolar bone consist of two parts.

a. cortical plates.

b. spongy bone.

Cortical plates: Consist of compact bone and forms the outer and inner plates of the alveolar process. The cortical plates, continuous with the compact layers of maxillary and mandibular body, are generally much thinner in the maxilla, than in the mandible. In maxilla, the outer cortical plate is perforated by many small opening through which blood and lymph vessels pass. In the lower jaw, the cortical bone of the alveolar process is dense. In the region of anterior teeth of both jaws, the supporting bone usually is very thin. No spongy bone is found here, and the cortical plate is fused with the alveolar bone proper. In such areas, notably in premolar and molar regions of the maxilla, defects of the outer alveolar wall are fairly common. Such defects, where periodontal tissues and covering mucosa fuse, do not impair the firm attachment and function of the tooth.

Spongy bone: Spongy bone fills the area between the cortical plate and the alveolar bone proper.

Age changes in bone: Periodontitis is commonly seen in older age and this resulting in the bone loss. Dental plaque and calculus play major role in development of periodontitis and subsequent bone loss.

Resorption after tooth loss follow a predictable pattern. The labial aspect of the alveolar crest is the principal site of resorption, with reduction first in width and later in height. The pattern of resorption is different in the maxilla and mandible. The residual alveolar ridge resorbs downwards and outwards in mandible, whereas in the maxilla the resorption is upwards and inwards.

The cause for resorption of alveolar bone after tooth loss has been assumed to be due to disease atrophy decreased blood localized inflammation or unfavorable prosthesis pressure.

Osteoporosis adversely affects collagen metabolism and bone mineralization, with concomitant decrease in bone mass. Severe osteoporosis reduces the bone mineral content of jaws and that may be associated with greater periodontal attachment loss and tooth loss. Oestrogen replacement for treatment for osteoporosis in older women has been associated with less gingival bleeding and may be beneficial in preventing tooth loss in postmenopausal women.

3

Oral Mucosa

ORAL MUCOUS MEMBRANE

The body cavities that communicate with the external surface are lined by mucous membrane, which are coated by serous and mucous secretions. The surface of oral cavity is a mucous membrane. Oral mucosa is continuous with skin of lip by vermilion border and posteriorly with mucosa of the pharynx.

Classification of Oral Mucosa

Based on the function, oral mucosa can be divided into three major types:

1. *Masticatory mucosa:* Gingiva and hard palate
2. *Lining or reflecting mucosa:* Lip, cheek, vestibular fornix, alveolar mucosa, floor of mouth and soft palate
3. *Specialized mucosa:* Dorsum of tongue and the taste buds

Masticatory mucosa is bound to bone and does not stretch. It bears forces generated when food is chewed. Lining mucosa covers the musculature and is distensible, adapting itself to the contraction and relaxation of cheeks, lips and tongue and to movements of the mandible produced by the muscles of mastication. Lining mucosa makes up all the surfaces of the mouth except for the dorsum of the tongue and masticatory mucosa. The specialized (sensory) mucosa is so called because it bears the taste buds, which have a sensory function.

Oral mucosa consists of:

- Epithelium
- Connective tissue (lamina propria)

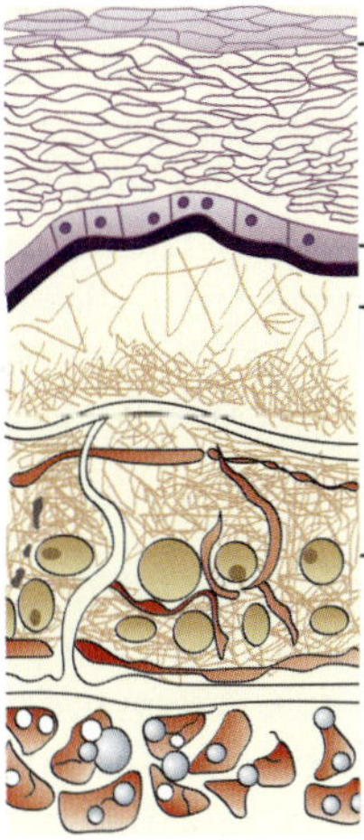

Fig. 3.1

It is attached by a loose connective tissue termed sub-mucosa to the underlying structure which may be bone or muscle.

Epithelium

Oral mucosal epithelium depending on the region may be nonkeratinised and if keratinized may be ortho or parakeratinized. The two layers, epithelium and connective tissue form an interface that is folded into corrugations. Papillae of connective tissue protrude toward the epithelium carrying the blood vessels and nerves. The epithelium in turn is formed into ridges that protrude toward the lamina propria. These ridges interdigitate with the papillae and are called epithelial ridges.

The epithelium and connective tissue are intimately connected. At their junction there are two different structures with very similar names, the basal lamina and basement membrane. The basal lamina is evident at the electron microscopic level and is epithelial in origin. The basement membrane is evident at the light microscopic level.

Basement Membrane

It is a zone that is 1 to 4 μm wide and is cell free. This zone stains positively with the periodic acid-schiff method, indicating that it contains neutral mucopolysaccharides. Ultrastructurally, basement membrane is called basal lamina, it is a basal complex consisting of lamina and fibers. The basal lamina is made up of a clear zone (lamina lucida) just below the epithelial cells and a dark zone (lamina densa) adjacent to the connective tissue. Anchoring fibrils, which contain type VII collagen, forms loops and are inserted into the lamina densa. Collagen fibres of type I and II run through these loops.

Lamina Propria

Lamina propria is connective tissue of variable thickness that supports the epithelium. It is divided into two parts—papillary and reticular. The papillary portion is between the epithelial ridges and reticular portion is below it. The reticular layer contains net like arrangement of collagen fibers. The lamina propria may attach to the periosteum of the alveolar bone, or it may overlay the submucosa, which varies in different regions of the mouth.

Submucosa

The submucosa consists of connective tissue of varying thickness and density. It attaches the mucous membrane to the underlying structures. Whether this attachment is loose or firm depends on the character of the submucosa. Glands, blood vessels, nerves and also adipose tissue are present in this layer. Compared to skin blood supply to oral mucosa is profuse and among the various regions blood flow to the gingiva is greatest. Submucosa may be present or absent. Looseness or density of its texture determines whether the mucous membrane is movably of immovably attached to the deeper layers.

Gingival Sulcus

The gingival sulcus or crevice is the space between the inner aspect of gingiva and the tooth. It is a continuous space present all around the tooth. The sulcus extends from the free gingival margin to the dentogingival junction. The sulcus may be responsible for the formation of the groove since it leaves the gingival margin without firm support. The sulcular (crevicular) epithelium is non-keratinized in humans. The sulcular epithelium is continuous with the gingival epithelium and the attachment epithelium. Under normal conditions the depth of the sulcus is variable; the average sulcus is 1.8 mm. Its depth increases due to periodontal diseases. Such a deepened gingival sulcus is periodontal pocket.

Dentogingival Junction

The junction between the gingiva and the tooth is dentogingival junction. The epithelium of gingiva which gets attached to the tooth is called junctional or attachment epithelium. The union between this epithelium and tooth is referred to as epithelial attachment. The junctional epithelium is best regarded as non-differentiating, non-keratinizing tissue lacking a gradient of change in cell types such as present in the gingival epithelium. Junctional epithelium extends up to 2 mm on the surface of the tooth. It has highest turnover rate of 5–6 days and therefore regenerates readily. The junctional epithelium is highly permeable and it has large intercellular spaces. It also permits easy flow of crevicular fluid. The junction of gingiva and the tooth is unique in many ways and may be a point of lessened resistance to mechanical forces and bacterial attack. The gingiva consists of two tissues maintaining the junction intact.

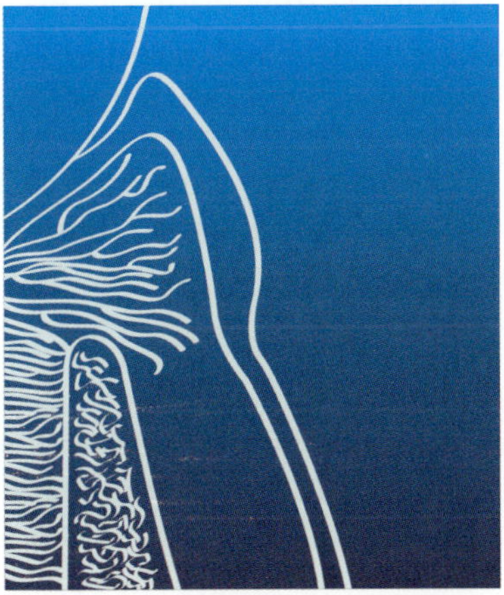

Fig. 3.2: Dentogingival junction

Shift of Dentogingival Junction

The position of the gingiva on the surface of the tooth changes with time. When the tip of the enamel first emerges through the mucous membrane of the oral cavity, the epithelium covers almost the entire enamel. The attachment epithelium separates from the enamel surface gradually while the crown emerges into the oral cavity.

At first after the tip of crown has appeared in the oral cavity, the epithelium separates rapidly from the surface of the tooth. Later, when the tooth comes to occlude with its antagonist, the separation of the attachment from the surface of the tooth slows down. When the tooth first reaches the plane of occlusion one-third to one-fourth of the enamel still remains covered by the gingiva.

The actual movement of the teeth toward the occlusal plane is termed active eruption. This applies to preclinical phase of eruption also. The separation of primary attachment epithelium from the enamel is termed passive eruption. The replacement of primary attachment epithelium by cells derived from the gingival epithelium is called secondary attachment epithelium.

There is a conceptual construct, called passive eruption that may be useful in describing the various levels of attachment that may occur as the gingiva recedes on the cementum. Some persons believe passive eruption to be a normal occurrence with aging. The belief that this is a 'normal' occurrence is probably incorrect. Crown exposure involving passive eruption and further recession has been described in four stages. The first two may be physiologic. Many conceive of the last two as normal also, but they are probably pathologic.

First stage: The bottom of the gingival sulcus remains in the region of the enamel-covered crown for some time, and the apical end of the attachment epithelium (reduced enamel epithelium) stays at the cementoenamel junction. This relation persists in primary teeth almost upto 1 year of age before shedding and in permanent teeth, usually to the age of 20 and 30 years. However, this relation is subject to a wide range of variation.

Second stage: The bottom of the gingival sulcus is still on the enamel, and the apical end of the attachment epithelium has shifted to the surface of the cementum.

The down growth of the attachment epithelium along the cementum is but one facet of the shift of the dentogingival junction. This entails dissolution of the fiber bundles that were anchored in the cervical parts of the cementum, now covered by the epithelium, and an apical shift of the gingival and transseptal fibers. The destruction of the fibers may be caused by enzymes formed by the epithelial cells, by plaque metabolites or enzymes, or by immunologic reactions as manifestations of periodontal disease. This stage of tooth exposure may persist to the age of 40 years or later.

Third stage: When the bottom of the gingival sulcus is at the cementoenamel junction, the epithelium attachment is entirely on the cementum, and the enamel-covered crown is fully exposed. This stage in the exposure of a tooth no longer is a passive manifestation. The epithelium shifts along the surface of the tooth and does not remain at the cementoenamel junction. This discontinuous and slow process is regarded as the body's attempt to maintain an intact dentogingival junction in the face of factors that cause its deterioration.

Fourth stage: The fourth stage represents recession of the gingiva. When the entire attachment is on cementum, the gingiva may appear normal but is believed to have receded as a result of pathology. It may occur without other clinical evidence of inflammatory periodontal disease.

The rates of crown exposure and recession vary in different persons. In some cases the fourth stage is observed in persons during their twenties. In other, even at 50 years of age of older the teeth are still in the first or second stage. The rate varies also in different teeth of the same jaw and on different surfaces of the same tooth. One side may be in the first stage and the other in the second or even the fourth stage.

The part of the tooth covered by enamel is the anatomic crown. The clinical crown is the part of the tooth exposed in the oral cavity. In the first and second stages the clinical crown is smaller than the anatomic crown. With recession (third stage) the entire enamel-covered part of the tooth is exposed, and the clinical crown is equal to the anatomic crown. Later the clinical crown is larger than the anatomic crown because parts of the root have been exposed (fourth stage). This type of crown exposure is to be produced by periodontal disease, loss of attachment (bone) and pocket formation

Age Changes in Oral Mucosa

With age the oral mucosa becomes smooth and dry. Histologically age related change are epithelial thinning, less prominent rete pegs, decreased cellular proliferation loss of submucosal elastin and fat and increased fibrotic connective tissues with degenerative alteration in collagen. Clinically these structural changes may be accompanied by dry thin smooth mucosal surfaces, with loss of elasticity and stippling. These changes may predispose the oral mucosa to trauma and infection, particularly when they are associated with denture use and salivary hypofunction. The filiform papilla becomes reduced and the tongue appears smooth owing to the reduction in the thickness of the epithelium. Nutritional deficiencies may also be a contributing factor for this change. Varicose veins on the ventral aspect of tongue are often seen and these are termed as lingual varies. Ectopic sebaceous gland (Fordyce's spots) is seen commonly in the elderly.

Older adults complains of diminished food recognition and also altered taste sensation. Age and oral and systemic disorders and their treatments can adversely affect taste function, which could place an older adult at risk for developing nutritional deficits and could adversely affect his or her quality of life.

4

Salivary Glands

The salivary glands are a group of compound exocrine glands secreting saliva. Saliva is a complex fluid produced by the salivary glands. The saliva forms a film of fluid coating the teeth and mucosa thereby creating and regulating a healthy environment in the oral cavity.

The parenchymal elements are derived from oral epithelium and consist of terminal secretory units leading into ducts that eventually open into the oval cavity. The connective tissue forms a capsule around the gland and ducts into lobes and lobules. The blood and lymph vessels and nerves that apply the gland are contained within that supply the glands are contained within the connective tissue.

The salivary glands are compound glands as they have more than are tubule entering the main duct. A duct is a passage that allows the glandular secretion emptied directly into an anatomic location where the secretion is to be used. The architectural arrangement of the salivary glands is tubuloacinar, where acini are secretory units.

Classification of Salivary Glands

- *Based on size and location*: Major and minor salivary glands
- *Histochemical nature of secretory products:* Serous and mucous

Structure of Terminal Secretory Units

The basic functional unit of a salivary gland is the terminal secretory unit called acini. The terminal secretory unit irrespective of size and location is made up of epithelial secretory cells, namely serous and mucous cells. The serous, mucous along with

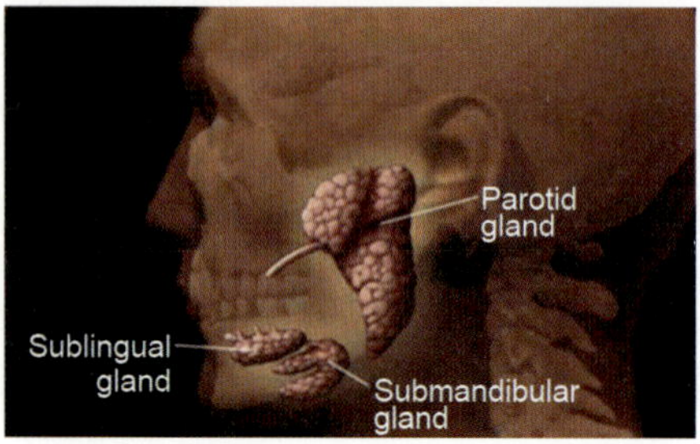

Fig. 4.1: Major salivary glands

myoepithelial cells are arranged in an acinus (or) acini (multiple) with a roughly spherical or tubular shape and a central lumen.

The cells in the acini rest on a basement membrane. They are arranged in a single layer. The intercellular spaces of the apical ends of the cells are separated from the lumen by junction complexes which are tight (zonula occludens), intermediate junction (zonula adherens) and are more desmosomes (macula adherens). The junctional complex hold the cells together in a acinus and regulate the permeability. The myoepithelial cells are located on the surface of the acini.

The central lumen of each acini may have a star shaped morphology because of extensions of lumen in between the cells called intercellular canaliculi the central lumen of the acini continue through a fine series of tubes which constantly merges with each other and grown larger eventually to merge into the main excretory duct. These tubes comprise of the ductal system.

Serous Cells

Serous secretory cells are pyramidal with a broad base on the basement membrane, the apex faces the lumen. The serous cells have a spherical nucleus placed at the basal region. The apical cytoplasms of these cells show accumulation of secretory granules. The granules are zymogen granules and are formed by glycolated proteins which are released into a vacuole.

Mucous Cells

The mucous cell, like the serous cell, is specialized for the synthesis, storage, and secretion of a secretory product. Its structure differs from that of serous cell. The nucleus and thin rim of cytoplasm are compressed against the base of the cell. Mucous cell shows accumulation of large amount of secretory product at the apical cytoplasm. The nucleus of mucous cell is oval or flattened in shape and located just above the basal plasma membrane.

Ducts

The ductal system of salivary glands consists of hollow tubes connected initially with the acinus and then with other ducts as the ducts progressively grown larger from the inner to outer portion of the gland each type of duct is lined by different type so epithelium, depending on its location in the gland. The ductal system is not just a pipeline or conduct for passageway for the saliva; it also actively participates in the production and modification of saliva. The three classes of ducts are intercalated, striated and excretory, each with differing structure and function.

Intercalated Ducts

The primary saliva produced by secreting end pieces passes first through the intercalated ducts. The lumen of end piece is continuous with the lumen of intercalated duct. Several ducts draining individual end pieces join to form larger intercalated ducts and these may join again before emptying into the striated ducts.

Striated Ducts

The striated ducts, which receive the primary saliva from the intercalated ducts, constitute the largest portion of the duct system. They are the main ductal component located within the lobules of the gland that is intralobular. The lumen is larger than those of secretory end pieces and intercalated ducts. An important function of striated duct cells is modification of primary saliva by reabsorption and secretion of electrolytes.

Excretory Ducts

The excretory ducts are located in the connective tissues septa between the lobules of the gland that is in extralobular or interlobular location. They are larger in diameter than striated ducts and have a pseudostratified columnar epithelium cells. In larger ducts occasional goblet cells and ciliated cells may be present. The ductal epithelium slowly undergoes a transition to striated, cuboidal and finally into stratified squamous epithelium when it merges with epithelium of oral cavity.

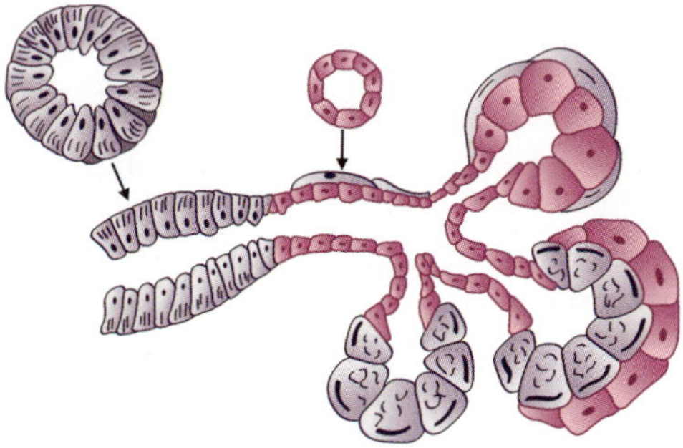

Fig. 4.2

Age Changes in Salivary Gland

With age a generalized loss of salivary gland parenchyma tissue occurs. The lost salivary cells often are replaced by adipose tissue. Although decreased production of saliva often is observed in older persons, whether this is related directly to the reduction in parenchymal tissue is not clear. Some studies of healthy older individuals, in which the use of medication were carefully controlled, revealed little or no loss of salivary function. Other studies suggest that although resting (unstimulated) salivary secretion is in the normal range, the volume of saliva produced during stimulated secretion is less than normal.

Older adults complains of diminished food recognition and also altered taste sensation. Age and oral and systemic disorders and their treatments can adversely affect taste function, which could place an older adult at risk for developing nutritional deficits and could adversely affect his/her quality of life.

Antibiotic prophylaxis should be considered for all patients with valvular heart disease.

Oral procedures and need for antibiotic prophylaxis to minimize risk of bacterial endocarditis.

5

Temporomandibular Joint

The articulation of the lower jaw with the cranium and upper facial skeleton involves two separate joints and the teeth when in occlusion. The joint although anatomically distinct, function in union and independent movements are not possible.

The temporomandibular articulation is a synovial joint. In human being the masticatory process demands the mandible to be capable not only of opening and closing movement but also of protrusive, retrusive and lateral movements but also of protrusive, retrusive and lateral movements and combinations. To achieve them the condyle undertakes translatory and rotary movements.

BONES OF THE JOINT

The bones of temporomandibular articulation are the glenoid fossa (an undersurface of squamous part of the temporal bone) and the

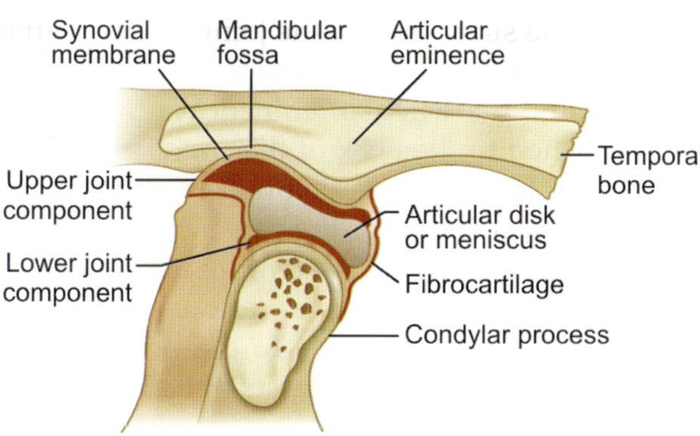

Fig. 5.1

condyle (supported by the condylar process of the mandible). Anteriorly glenoid fossa is bounded by a ridge of bone described as articular eminence, which also is involved in the articulation. The middle part is a thin plate of bone of the upper surface of which forms the middle cranial fossa (housing the temporal lobe of the brain).

The condyle is the articulating surface of the mandible. Unlike most synovial joints, the articular surfaces of which are covered with hyaline cartilage. This histologic distinction has been used to argue that the TMJ is not a weight-bearing joint, but the reality for this distinction can be found in the developmental history of the joint.

The glenoid fossa always is covered by a thin fibrous layer that directly overlies the bone, much as periosteum does but this layer becomes appreciably thick where it covers the slope of the articular eminence.

Capsule, Ligaments and Disk of the Joint

The capsule of a synovial joint is an important structure. The capsule consists of dense collagenous membrane that seals the joint space and provides passive stability enhanced by increased local thickenings in its walls to from anatomically recognizable ligaments, as well as active stability from proprioceptive nerve endings in the capsule

Extension of the fibrous capsule into the joint cavity form disks that function as articular surfaces and divide the joint into two compartments. Recognizing the disk as an extension of the capsule, the capsule of TMJ can be described as a fibrous non-elastic membrane surrounding the joint which is attached above to the squamotympanic fissure posteriorly, the margins of glenoid fossa laterally and the articular eminence anteriorly inferiorly the capsule is attached to the neck of the condyle above the disk the capsule is fairly lax, whereas below it is tightly attached to the condyle. The lateral aspect of the capsule is thickened to form a fan-shaped ligament know as temporomandibular ligament, which runs obliquely backward and downward from the lateral aspect of the articular eminence to the posterior aspect of the condylar neck. The ligament consists of two parts:

1. An outer oblique portion arising from the outer surface of the articular eminence and extending backward and downward to insert into the outer surface of the condylar neck.
2. An inner horizontal portion with the same origin but inserting into the lateral pole of the condyle.

The capsule and its lateral thickening form the ligament of the joint. Joint ligaments restrict and limit the distance that the bones forming the articulation can be separated from each other without causing tissue damage. The temporomandibular ligament restricts, displacements of the mandible in three different planes. First, the ligament functions in a way similar to collateral ligaments of other joints because of the bilateral nature of the articulation. By preventing lateral dislocation of one joint, it prevents medial dislocation of the other. Second, its oblique component limits the amount of inferior displacement, and third, its horizontal component prevents or limits posterior displacement.

Two other ligaments are included in conventional descriptions of the joint, although neither has a function and the first, is the sphenomandibular ligament running from the lingual and shielding the opening of the inferior alveolar canal to the spine of the sphenoid. The second is the stylomandibular ligament, running from the spine of the sphenoid to the angle of mandible.

An inward circumferential extension of the capsule forms a tongue, fibrous disk that divides the joint into upper and lower compartments, provides an articular surface for head of the condyle and because the lower half of the capsule is tightly bound to the condyle, moves with the condyle during translation. The disk consists of dense fibrous tissue and its shape conforms to that of the apposed articular surfaces.

The lower surface of the disk is concave surface because its posterior and anterior components are considerably thickened; delimiting a central thinner component at rest, this central thinner component of the disk separates the anterior eminence. The thickened posterior portion occupies the gap between the condyle and the floor of the glenoid fossa, and the anterior portion lies slightly anterior to the condyle.

The anterior portion of the disk fuses with the anterior wall of capsule. Above the point of fusion, the capsule runs forward to blend with the periosteum of the anterior slope of articular eminence below, the capsule merges with the periosteum of the front of the neck of the condyle. Posteriorly, the disk also appears to divide into two lamellae, but again these lamellae represent the posterior wall of the capsule. The upper part of the capsule or lamella consists of fibrous and elastic tissue and inserts into the squamotympanic fissure. The lower part of the capsule, the upper part of the capsule or lamellae, consists of fibrous and elastic tissue and inserts into the squamotympanic fissure. The lower part of the capsule, consisting of collagen only and nonelastic, blends with the periosteum of the condylar neck. Between these two lamellae a space is created that is filled with a loose, highly vascular connective tissue. The disk is well supplied with vascular and neural elements at its periphery but is avascular and not innervated in its central region.

Synovial Membrane

The capsule is lined in its inner surface by a synovial membrane is considered to line the entire capsule, with folds or villi of the membrane protruding into the joint cavity, especially in its fornices and its upper posterior aspect. The synovial membrane does not cover the articular surfaces of the joint or the disk, except for its bilaminar posterior region.

Muscles of Mastication

The muscles of mastication are the masseter, medial (inferior) pterygoid, lateral (superior) pterygoid and the temporalis. In functional terms, other muscle groups are involved in mastication, such as the posterior group (which stabilizes the cranial base) and the infrahyoid group (which stabilizes the hyoid bone and permits the mylohyoid muscle and anterior belly of the digastric muscle to influence mandibular position).

The masseter and medial pterygoid muscles together have a sling-like configuration clasping the angle of the mandible and are the principal elevators of the jaw. The temporalis muscle-anterior fibers act as an elevator and its posterior horizontally disposed fibers acts as retractor of the mandible. The lateral pterygoid muscle has two heads, superior head, and inferior head

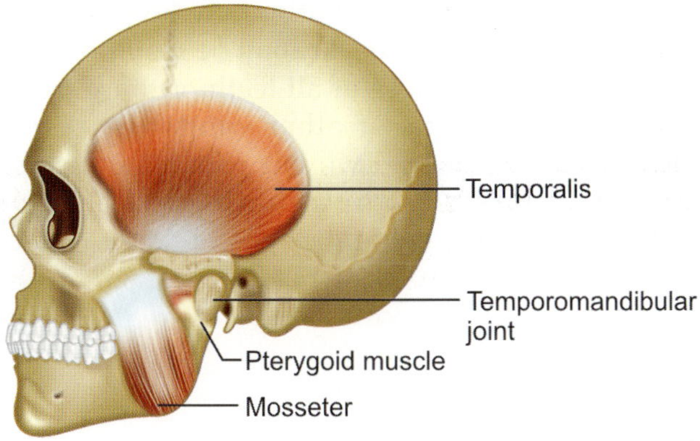

Fig. 5.2

and on contraction they bring about downward-forward and medial movement of the condyle.

Age Change in Temporomandibular Joint

After the loss of posterior teeth, change in the force or direction of stress may cause structural changes. These changes may include fibrillation (separation between collagen bundles) of the fibrous covering of the articulating surface of the disk. Abnormal functional activities may also produce injury to the articular bones. Compensation and partial repair may be accomplished by the development of cartilage on the condylar surface and in the disk.

The articular surface is capable of remodeling due to functional demands. It shows changes due to loss of teeth or due to attrition of teeth. The folds in synovial membrane increases in number, with age and are also more prominent in joints affected by a pathologic process.

Osteoarthritis (Degenerative Joint Disease)

Osteoarthritis develop in persons past 40 years of age. Although its etiology is not known, it is a disease associated with the aging process.

Osteoarthritis first involves the weight bearing bones of the body since TMJ is not a weight bearing joint, changes here are insignificant even though arthropathy may be present in other joints. Those changes that do occur may be result of distributed balance of the joint due to loss of all teeth or to external injury. Patients with osteoarthritis of other joints may complain of clicking and snapping in the TMJ, but pain is not necessarily a feature. This joint noise is probably due to atypical disk motion resulting from disordered mandibular condyle disk function on the basis of the changes in the articular cartilage limitation of motion or ankylosis rarely occurs.

Section II

Oral Considerations in Systemic Disease Associated with Old Age

6

Gastrointestinal Diseases

GASTROINTESTINAL TRACT

Gastroesophageal Reflux Disease

Gastroesophageal reflux disease is one of the commonly occurring diseases affecting the upper gastrointestinal tract. During gastroesophageal reflux, gastric contents passively move up from the stomach into esophagus. While this may occur normally, it may be attributed to GERD if it is associated with symptoms. The symptoms of GERD can be quite varied; they are primarily symptoms that are associated with the sequelae of mucosal injury. These resultant injuries include esophagitis, esophageal ulceration, stricture, and dysplasia. Chest pain is another important symptom that is related to disorders of oesophagus. Chest pain can mimic the symptoms of an acute cardiovascular disorder.

Dysphagia is also a common complaint present.

Oral Considerations

Patients who experience GERD complain of dysgeusia (foul taste), dental sensitivity, erosion, and/or pulpitis. Dental sensitivity is due to erosion of enamel by gastric acid. Erosion leads to dentin sensitivity and at times irreversible pulp involvement. Patients who have a diagnosis of GERD may need to be treated in a semisupine position and premedicated with H_2 receptor antagonists or antacids. Any medications that may cause nausea should be prescribed judiciously because of increased likelihood of regurgitation and possible aspiration. Sodium bicarbonate rinse to minimize dysgeusia due to acid reflux. Topical fluoride applications will ensure optimal dental mineralization. Oral mucosa changes such as erythema and mucosa atrophy may be present as a result of the exposure of tissues to acid.

Hiatal Hernia

The Oesophagus passes through the diaphragmatic hiatus and into stomach just inferior to the diaphragm. The incidence of hiatal hernia increases with age although the condition is also seen in infants and children.

Symptoms of hiatal hernia include chest pain, which may radiate in patterns similar to those of myocardial infarction pain. Adult patients with hiatal hernia may experience reflux into the oesophagus. Chronic gastrointestinal reflux can erode the oesophageal lining, causing bleeding, which may lead to anemia. Chronic oesophageal inflammation may produce scarring, resulting in oesophageal narrowing.

Oral Considerations

If a hiatal hernia is treated with medication that causes xerostomia, the dose and drug type may need to be altered by the patient's physician. Dry mouth may be treated by artificial saliva, alcohol free mouth washes or increased fluid intake.

Peptic Ulcer

Peptic ulcer disease is common benign ulceration of epithelial lining of the stomach (gastric ulcer) or duodenum (duodenal ulcer).

Peptic ulcer disease includes both gastric ulcers and duodenal ulcers. Increasing use of NSAIDs has inherent damaging effects on the gastroduodenal mucosa. The gastric ulcers primarily resulted from altered with increase acid production. *Helicobacter pyroli* plays a vital role in peptic ulcer development in both sites.

Most patients with the disease have recurrent pain and consult their physician to relief of symptoms and to prevent recurrence. Life threatening complications are hemorrhage, perforation or obstruction. It is essential that dentists 1) recognize the morbidity associated with peptic ulcers and the symptoms associated with undiagnosed or poorly managed peptic ulcer disease, 2) make a referral to the primary care physician or gastroenterologist when these symptoms are recognized.

Gastric Ulcer

Gastric ulcers occur more often after 50 years of age. Gastric ulcers present with epigastric pain radiating to the back. Pain is aggravated by food. Standard medical treatment of gastric ulcers involves antacid components, antibiotics to eradicate *H. pylori* and H_2 blocking agents.

Duodenal Ulcer

Duodenal ulcer represents a break through the mucosa into the submucosa or deeper. The base of the ulcer is necrotic tissue consisting of pus and fibrin. When the ulcer erodes into an adjacent blood vessel, there is hemorrhage. If erosion continues through the serous outer layer of duodenum adjacent organs or perforation into the peritoneal cavity occurs. When conditions are favorable the ulcer heals, with granulation tissue and new epithelium. If ulcer is present for prolonged periods, it becomes associated with scar tissue and possible deformity.

Most common symptom of an uncomplicated ulcer is epigastric pain. The pain is often perceived as a burning or gnawing sensation sometimes associated with nausea and vomiting and usually occurs when stomach is empty to adequately buffer the acid stimulated by the meal. Therefore, the pain begins one or more hours after eating and when the patient is asleep.

Oral Considerations

Dental erosion in the palatal aspect of the maxillary teeth is seen due to persistent regurgitation of gastric acid. Vascular malformations of the lip have been reported and range from a very small macule to a large venous pool. To present aggravation of the disease, the avoidance of actions that increase the production of acid is essential.

Lengthy procedures should be avoided. Drugs exacerbating ulceration such as NSAIDs and acetaminophen products should be avoided. Patients taking anticholinergic drugs present xerostomia and this may be particularly problematic for denture wearers. Denture adhesives and artificial saliva may aid in the retention of this prosthesis. Before extensive oral surgical or periodontal procedures are undertaken, it is essential to determine

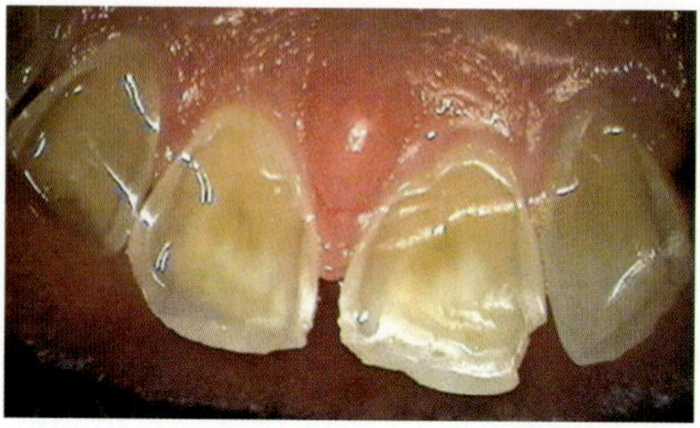

Fig. 6.1: Dental erosion in the palatal aspect

the patient's oral red blood cell count, hemoglobin, hematocrit and platelet count. If the patient has a history of ulcer perforation and subsequent hemorrhage, blood loss can result in anemia. Associated risks of anemia are as delayed healing, bacterial infection, and grave side effects of respiratory depression by narcotic analgesics enhanced by a state of anemia. Cimetidine and ranitidine drugs commonly prescribed for duodenal ulcer patients have occasionally been associated with thrombocytopenia.

7

Respiratory Diseases

ASTHMA

Asthma is a chronic disease that affects the lower airways. It is characterized by recurrent and reversible airflow limitation due to an underlying inflammatory process.

Etiology

The etiology of asthma is unknown but allergic sensitivity is seen in most patients with asthma. Genetic factors may play a role, but no single gene or combination of genes has been identified.

Clinical Findings

The clinical features of asthma are recurrent reversible airflow limitation and airway hyper responsiveness. These factors lead to the development of the signs and symptoms of asthma, which include intermittent wheezing, coughing, dyspnea and chest tightness. Symptoms of asthma tend to worsen at night and in the early morning hours. Triggers are allergens, exercise, cold air, respiratory irritants, emotional extremes and infections (especially viral infections). Symptoms can progress slowly over time or they may develop abruptly.

Chronic coughing with nocturnal awakenings, dyspnea or chest tightness with exertion, recurrent bronchitis associated with infections of upper respiratory tract and wheezing that occurs on seasonal basis. Common findings in more severe disease include an increased anteroposterior chest diameter, a prolonged expiratory phase, wheezing and diminished breath sounds. Digital clubbing is rarely seen. Concurrent allergic disease such as allergic rhinitis may be present. During acute exacerbations, patients may show signs of respiratory distress, with tachypnea, intercostal retractions, nasal flaring and cyanosis.

Management

Pharmacotherapy of asthma is based on the severity of disease. Patients with mild-intermittent disease usually require shortacting bronchodilators. These medications (albuterol) are preferably administered by inhalation. Patients with mild persistent asthma require routine therapy for control of underlying airway inflammation. Inhaled corticosteroids are most effective asthma anti-inflammatory agents.

Oral Considerations

The main concern when treating any medically compromised patient is to avoid exacerbation of the underlying condition.

Numerous dental products and materials, including toothpaste, fissure sealants, tooth enamel dust and methyl methacrylate have been associated with the exacerbation of asthma whereas fluoride trays and rolls are suggested as being so associated.

Oral manifestations include candidiasis, decreased salivary flow, increased calculus, increased gingivitis, increased periodontal disease, and increased incidence of caries and adverse effects of orthodontic therapy.

Prolonged use of β_2 agonists may cause reduced salivary flow, with a resulting increase in cariogenic bacteria and caries and an increased incidence of candidiasis.

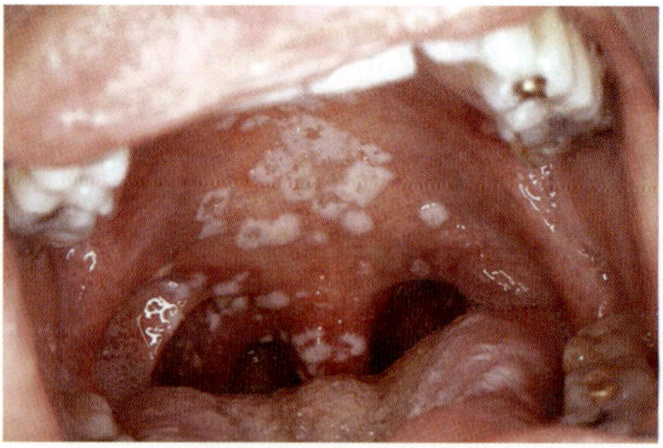

Fig. 7.1: Oral candidiasis

Electric dental procedures should be avoided in all but those whose asthma is well controlled.

Recommendations for administering dental care to patients who have asthma:

- Fluoride supplements instituted for all asthmatic patients particularly those taking β_2 agonists.
- Rinsing mouth after using inhalers.
- Oral hygiene reinforced to reduce the incidence of gingivitis and periodontitis.
- Antifungal medications should be administered as needed, particularly in patients who are taking inhaled corticosteroids.
- Barbiturates and narcotics should be avoided due to their potential to cause bronchospasm and reduce respiratory functions.
- Avoid dental materials they may precipitate an attack. Acrylic appliances should be cured prior to insertion. Dental materials without methyl methacrylate should be considered.
- Schedule appointments for late mornings and later in the day, to minimize risk of an asthmatic attack.
- Have oxygen and bronchodilators available in case of an exacerbation of asthma.
- There are no contraindications to the use of oral anaesthetics containing epinephrine, but preservatives such as sodium metabisulfite may contribute to asthma exacerbation in susceptible patients. Interactions between epinephrine and β_2 agonists may result in a synergistic effect, producing increased blood pressure and arrhythmias.
- Judicious use of rubber dam will present reduced breathing capability.
- Up to 10% of adult asthmatic patients have an allergy to aspirin and other non-steriodal anti-inflammatory agents. Although use of acetaminophen has been proposed as an alternative to use of aspirin, recent data suggest caution because these type of drugs have also been associated with more severe asthma.

- During an acute asthmatic attack, discontinue the dental procedure, remove all intraoral device, place the patient in a comfortable position, make sure the airway is opened and administer a β_2 agonists and oxygen. If no improvement is noted, administer epinephrine subcutaneously (1:1,000 concentration, 0.01 mg/kg of body weight, up to a maximum of 0.3 mg) and alert emergency medical assistance.

CHRONIC OBSTRUCTIVE PULMONARY DISEASE (COPD)

Chronic obstructive pulmonary disease is a term used to describe chronic and largely irreversible airway obstruction due to inflammation of lower airways. Chronic bronchitis in COPD is due to chronic bronchial inflammation. Chronic bronchitis is diagnosed on clinical criteria and is defined as coughing and sputum production for 3 or more months per year for atleast 2 consecutive years. Dyspnea and hypoxemia are features of COPD.

Clinical Findings

The clinical course of patients with COPD is quite varied. Most patients display some degree of progressive dyspnea, exercise intolerance and fatigue. Patients are susceptible to frequent exacerbations, usually caused by infections of the upper and lower respiratory tract. Patients with chronic bronchitis present with dyspnea, cough and sputum production. An increase in production of often purulent sputum is a sign of exacerbation due to respiratory infections. Physical findings include diffuse wheezing, possibly associated with signs of respiratory distress including the use of accessory muscles of respiration and tachypnea.

Management

There are no curative treatments for chronic bronchitis and emphysema. Management focuses on maintaining quality of life and presenting exacerbations. Maintenance therapy includes inhaled bronchodilators such as albuterol and ipratropium bromide. Oxygen administration to be used with caution in COPD patients as their ventilator drive will be diminished. This is the result of chronic retention of carbondioxide and subsequent insensitivity to hypercapnia. As a result, patients with COPD are sensitive to increases in oxygen tension.

Prognosis is poor for patients who are frequently symptomatic due to COPD. The 5 years mortality rate is approximately 50%, with most patients dying from respiratory failure.

Oral Considerations

Associations between oral infections and COPD have been suggested by several epidemiologic studies. Periodontal pathogens have shown to be the causative pathogen of exacerbation in 4% of individuals with COPD. One prospective study suggested that oral colonization with respiratory pathogens in patients residing in a chronic care facility was significantly associated with COPD. It is essential that elderly individuals receive adequate oral hygiene in order to minimize respiratory complications.

As mentioned above, increased oxygen tension may diminish respiratory function in patients with COPD. Extreme caution must be exercised when administering supplemental oxygen in emergencies.

Pulmonary Embolism

Pulmonary embolism is defined as a blockage of a pulmonary arterial vessel due to thromboembolic event. The embolus may originate anywhere, but it is usually due to thrombosis in the lower extremities.

Risk factors for pulmonary embolism:

- Prolonged immobilization (such as in a postoperative state)
- History of deep-vein thrombosis
- Low-extremity trauma.

Clinical Findings

Patients usually present with dyspnea. Other features include chest pain, fever, diaphoresis, cough, hemoptysis and syncope. Physical findings can include evidence of a lower-extremity deep-vein thrombosis, tachypnea, crackles or rub on lung auscultation and heart murmur.

Management

Fibrinolytic agents such as streptokinase and urokinase are effective for rapid lysis of emboli. Newer fibrinolytic agents include tissue type plasminogen activator, single chain urokinase like plasminogen activator and antistreplase. A heparin infusion is started, followed by long-term management with warfarin. Surgical embolectomy can be performed in unstable patients from whom anticoagulants are contraindicated.

Prognosis

Although many patients with pulmonary embolism die before medical attention is received. The rate of mortality due to pulmonary embolism once adequate anticoagulation therapy is initiated is less than 5%.

Oral Considerations

The main concern in the provision of dental care for individuals with pulmonary embolism is the patient who is being managed with oral anticoagulants. As a general rule, dental care (including simple extractions) can safely be provided for patients with prothrombin time of up to 20 seconds or an international normalized ratio of 2.5. It is recommended that any dental care for these patients be coordinated with their primary medical care provider.

8

Cardiovascular Diseases

HYPERTENSION

Hypertension is defined as having systolic blood pressure ≥ 140 mm Hg or diastolic blood pressure ≥ 90 mm Hg or as having to use anti-hypertensive medications.

Etiology

Hypertension is classified as primary (essential) and secondary. Ninety-five percent of all hypertension is of unknown cause. There are many secondary causes, but these account for only 5 to 10% of patients with hypertension. These include renal disorders such as renal parenchymal disease, renovascular disease, renin-producing tumors, and primary sodium retention. Endocrinologic disturbances that may result in hypertension include thyroid disease, adrenal disorders and exogenous hormones.

Physical Examination

The main goals of the physical examination are to look for signs of end-organ damage (such as retinopathy) and to find evidence of a cause of secondary hypertension. Thus the peripheral pulses should be auscultated for a renal artery bruit that would indicate renovascular hypertension. The presence of an upper abdominal diastolic bruit that localized toward one side is highly suggestive of renal artery stenosis. The physical examination should include a fundoscopic assessment.

Management

A large number of agents exists, including diuretics, β-blockers, calcium channel blockers, angiotensin-converting enzyme inhibitors, angiotensin II receptor blockers, direct vasodilators, and centrally acting agents.

Prognosis

Treatment of hypertension is important because it reduces overall mortality. Improved control of hypertension contributed to the decline in mortality from cardiovascular disease. Anti-hypertensive pharmacotherapy have its predominant effect on stroke mortality.

Oral Health Considerations

The patients with high blood pressure are at increased risk of adverse advents in a dental setting when target organ disease is present. However, the absence of target organ disease does not mitigate a careful evaluation and treatment of patients within safe and appropriate parameters of care.

Table 8.1: Common oral hypertensive medications

Drug	*Side effects*
Diuretics	• Increased cholesterol and glucose levels • Oral dryness
Adrenergic inhibitors	• Postural hypertension • Nasal congestion • Sedation • Bradycardia • Oral ulcerations • Oral dryness
Direct vasodilators	• Headaches • Tachycardia
Calcium antagonists	• Gingival overgrowth
ACE inhibitors	• Lichenoid reactions of the oral mucosa • Cough • Loss of taste

Blood pressure measurement in the dental setting

Routine blood pressure measurements

Measure and record at initial visit.

Recheck:

Every 2 years for patients with BP < 130/85.

Every year for patients with BP of 130 – 139/85 – 89.

Every visit for patients with BP ≥ 140/90.

Every visit for patients with diagnosed hypertension.

Before initiating dental care

Assess presence of hypertension.

Determine presence of target organ disease.

After checking BP, determine treatment modifications

Dental treatment for patients with elevated BP

Asymptomatic, BP < 159/99, no target organ disease.

No dental modifications needed

Can safely be treated in a dental outpatient setting

Asymptomatic, BP = 160 – 179/100 – 109, no history of target organ disease.

Assessment on individual basis with regard to type of dental procedure

BP ≥ 180/110, no history of target organ disease

No elective dental care

Target organ disease or poorly controlled diabetes mellitus.

Elective dental care only when BP is controlled, preferably < 140/90

CORONARY ARTERY DISEASE

Coronary artery disease accounts for approximately 30 to 50% of all cases of cardiovascular disease. Atherosclerosis, the most common causes of coronary artery disease, results from a wide variety of pathologic processes that interact with and disrupt the vascular endothelium. The result is plaque formation, with the compromise of effective arterial luminal area. In the coronary circulation, this process may cause a chronic reduction in coronary blood flow and ensuring myocardial ischemia or it may cause acute plaque rupture, with intracoronary thrombus formation and subsequent myocardial infarction. Atherosclerosis may affect any vascular bed, including the coronary, cerebral, renal, mesenteric and peripheral vascular systems. When endorgan blood flow is compromised, the resulting ischemia can cause subsequent organ dysfunction.

Etiology

Atherosclerosis is responsible for almost all cases of coronary artery disease. This insidious process begins with a fatty streak, first seen in early adolescence; these progress into plaques in early adulthood and may result in thrombotic occlusions and coronary events in middle age and later life.

Risk Factor

Lipids: The total cholesterol concentration in serum is a major and clearcut risk factor for coronary heart disease. The risk of coronary heart disease progressively increased with higher values of serum total cholesterol.

Hypertension is well established risk factors of adverse cardiovascular outcomes including coronary heart disease morbidity and mortality, stroke, coronary heart failure and sudden death

Glucose intolerance and diabetes mellitus: Insulin resistance, hyperinsulinemia and glucose intolerance all appear to promote atherosclerosis.

Cigarette smoking is important and potentially reversible risk factor for coronary heart disease and coronary heart disease events such as myocardial infarction. Risk increases with increasing tobacco consumption.

Estrogen deficiency: The incidence of coronary heart disease in women increases after menopause, an effect that is thought to be secondary to low serum levels of estrogen.

Lifestyle and dietary factors: Dietary factors such as high calorie, high fat and high cholesterol diet contribute to the development of other risk factors such as obesity, hyperlipidemia and diabetes that predispose to coronary heart disease. Increased intake of dietary fiber is associated with a decreased risk of coronary heart disease.

Exercise: Even a moderate degree of exercise appears to have a protective effect against coronary heart disease and all cause mortality.

Obesity: It is associated with the development of a number of risk factors of coronary heart disease, including systemic hypertension, impaired glucose metabolism, insulin resistance, hypertriglyceridemia, reduced HDL cholesterol and elevated fibrinogen.

Management

The management of coronary artery disease depends on a number of clinical factors, including the extent and severity of ischemia, exercise capacity, prognosis base on exercise testing, overall LV function and associated disease such as diabetes mellitus. Medical therapy includes the selected use of aspirin, β blockers, ACE inhibitors. These agents reduce the incidence and subsequent MI and death. Nitrates and calcium channels blockers may be added to the primary agents to relieve symptoms of ischemia in selected patients. Percutaneous coronary intervention with percutaneous transluminal coronary angioplasty and intracoronary stenting relieves symptoms of chronic ischemia, improves mortality when used acutely in patients with myocardial infarction, and improves regional or left ventricle function, specifically in patients with single vessel or multivessel coronary artery disease.

Oral Considerations

The primary concern for the dental provides is to prevent the recurrence of ischemia or infarction. The risk for such an event to take place is determined by numerous factors, including the underlying type of coronary artery disease (stable angina, MI). Furthermore, there is a temporal relationship between recurrences of ischemia events, which influences the risk for subsequent acute episodes. Impaired hemostasis also requires dental modifications. Side effects from cardiac drugs may cause oral changes, and drug interactions with medications used for dental care may occur.

General Precautions Regarding Dental Procedures

It is highly recommended that all dental professionals treating patients who have history of ischemic heart disease be versed in advanced cardiac life support (ACLS) or at least basic cardiac life support (BCLS).

The determination of vital signs prior to dental care is essential. Blood pressure and pulse rate and rhythm should be recorded. Most events occur between 6.00 am and noon. It has been proposed that sympathetic nervous system activation and an increased coagulative state may be precipitating factors. Medications that present these events such as β blockers, aspirin and antihypertensives should be continued. Dental care should therefore be provided in the late morning or the early afternoon.

Electric procedures, especially those requiring general anesthesia, should be avoided for atleast 4 weeks following acute myocardial infarction as there is a small increased risk of recurrent events.

Anticoagulation Therapy and Dental Care

Patients with coronary artery disease require the use of aspirin. Additional antiplatelet agents are also instituted after coronary artery stenting. Daily aspirin is continued at the conclusion of 4 week. These agents may increase the risk of bleeding when used in combination.

Anticoagulation therapy is used to treat and to present thromboembolism, and different types of medications are used to achieve anticoagulation, based on the patients underlying medical condition. Medical conditions for which prophylactic anticoagulation therapy is instituted include atrial fibrillation, valvular heart disease, cerebrovascular accidents, pulmonary embolism and deep-vein thrombosis.

Two major types of medications are used for anticoagulation:

1. Drugs with antiplatelet activity
2. Drugs with antithrombin activity.

Most common antiplatelet drug is aspirin, which is used chronically in very low doses to prevent cardiovascular and cerebrovascular events. Aspirin will irreversibly decrease platelet aggregation and consequently increase the bleeding time. If the patient has other underlying medical conditions that predispose to impaired homeostasis (such as uremia or liver disease), takes other anticoagulants (NSAIDs), abuse alcohol, aspirin should be discontinued 3 to 7 days prior to surgery.

If emergency surgery needs to be performed and the patient's bleeding time is higher than 15 to 20 minutes, 1-desamino-8-D-arginine vasopressin (DDAVP) can be instilled to improve homestasis. DDAVP is administered parenterally at 0.3 μg/kg of body weight with a maximum dose of 20 to 24 μg within 1 hour of surgery. There have been no studies indicating the need to discontinue and alter anticoagulation therapy prior to minor oral surgical procedures for patients taking other types of antiplatelet medications.

The most commonly used antithrombin medications are dicumarols (e.g. warfarin). The full therapeutic effect of warfarin is reached after 48 to 72 hours and will last for 36 to 72 hours if the drug is discontinued. The efficacy of warfarin therapy is monitored by the prothrombin time or the international normalized ratio (INR). The INR is calculated on the basis of international sensitivity index of the specific thromboplastin used in the test. The therapeutic level of the INR is dependent on the underlying condition but is usually kept at a range of from 2.0 to 4.5. For an accurate assessment of an individual's anticoagulation status, and INR calculation should be performed within 24 hours of surgery. There is little indication that anticoagulation therapy should be discontinued before minor oral surgical procedures when the patient's INR is < 3.0. This conclusion is based on the minimal increase of intraoral bleeding tendency at this level of anticoagulation and on the ease with which it is possible to stop most intraoral bleeding with local measures.

Three different protocols can be used to treat patients with significantly elevated INR.

1. First protocol
   - Warfarin is not discontinued.
   - This minimizes adverse thrombo-embolic events but increases the risk for excessive bleeding after surgery.

- If localized antihemostatic measures are inadequate to stop bleeding after surgery, vitamin K injection and anti-fibrinolytic mouth rinses instituted

2. Second protocol
   - Warfarin therapy is discontinued
   - Medication must be discontinued 2 to 3 days before surgery
   - It will take an additional 2 to 3 days after surgery to regain the therapeutic effect of the medication

     (During this time, the patient is at an increased risk for developing thrombo-embolic event but will not exhibit increased bleeding tendencies after surgery)
3. Third protocol
   - Warfarin therapy is discontinued and patient is placed on an alternative

     Anticoagulation therapy
   - The greatest advantage is that the patient's risk for developing thrombo-embolic events is minimized.
   - Heparin is continued until approximately 6 hours before surgery and is continued after surgery in combination with oral anticoagulation therapy until a desirable INR has been reached.

In addition, due to surgical procedure involved such patients may have insignificant pain when sitting in a dental chair, even several weeks after their heart surgery. Elective dental care should therefore be postponed until the patient can sit comfortable in dental chair.

Prosthetic Heart Valves

Prosthetic heart valves are either mechanical or bioprosthetic. Patients with mechanical valves are placed on anticoagulation therapy to prevent thromboembolism. Patients with mitral valve prothesis are at approximately twice the risk of those with aortic valve prothesis. The risk of thromboembolism is highest in the period following placement of the valve and decreases over time as the valve becomes endothelialized. Bioprosthetic valve have a lower thrombogenic potential and do not need to be accompanied by long-term anti-coagulation therapy.

Prosthetic heart valves increase the risk of infectious endocarditis, which typically manifests as fever and as other systemic symptoms.

Mitral Valve Disease

Mitral valve disease may occur in many form, including mitral valve prolapse, mitral regurgitation and mitral stenosis.

Mitral valve prolapse occurs as a result of myxomatous degeneration of mitral leaflets and supporting apparatus. This results in abnormal movement or prolapsed of the mitral leaflets posteriorly toward the left atrium during mechanical systole. A small percentage of those with mitral valve prolapsed have significant mitral regurgitation and ensuring left ventricular volume overload.

Mitral regurgitation occurs as a result of wide variety of abnormalities of the mitral leaflets. These abnormalities have various causes, including myxomatous degeneration and leaflet prolapsed, rheumatic heart disease, endocarditis and use of anorectic agents such as fenfluramine and phentermine.

Mitral stenosis most often occurs as a result of rheumatic heart disease or a congenital process. In rheumatic heart disease, there is characteristic thickening and fusion of the mitral commissures as well as thickening and calcification of the leaflets and subvalvular apparatus. This results in a restriction of left ventricular inflow, subsequent left atrial hypertension and enlargement, atrial arrhythmias and secondary pulmonary hypertension.

Oral Considerations

Antibiotic prophylaxis should be considered for all patients with valvular heart disease.

Oral procedures and need for antibiotic prophylaxis to minimize risk of bacterial endocarditis	
Oral procedures requiring antibiotic prophylaxis·	Oral procedures not requiring prophylaxis (clinical judgement - may indicate antibiotic prophyaxis with any procedure they may result in significant bleeding
• Extractions • Periodontal procedures: surgery subgingival placement of antibiotic fibers, scaling and root planning • Implant placement • Tooth reimplantation • Placement of orthodontic bands (not brackets) • Endodontic instrumentation or surgery (beyond apex) • Intraligamentary injections • Procedures in which significant bleeding is anticipated	• Operative and prosthodontic procedures (restorations and replacement of missing teeth • Nonligamentary local anaesthetic injections • Intracanal endodontic procedures • Placement of removable prosthodontic or orthodontic appliances • Orthodontic appliance adjustment • Impression taking • Oral radiograph • Fluoride treatment • Placement of rubber dams • Postoperative suture removal

Antibiotic prophylaxis to minimize risk of bacterial endocarditis after oral procedures	
Adults not allergic to penicillin	2 gm amoxicillin 1 hour before procedure (oral route) 2 gm ampicillin IM or IV within 30 minutes before procedure
Adults, penicillin allergic	1 hour before procedure (oral route) – 600 mg clindamycin, or – 2 gm cephalexin, or – 500 mg azithromycin 600 mg clindamycin (IV) – 30 minutes before procedure or

Contd.

Contd.

	1 gm cefazolin (IM/IV) – 30 minutes before procedure
Children, not allergic to penicillin	50 mg/kg amoxicillin – 1 hour before procedure (oral route) 50 mg/kg ampicillin – 30 minutes before procedure (oral route)
Children, penicillin allergic	Oral route 1 hour before procedure – 20 mg/kg clindamycin – 50 mg/kg cephalaxin – 15 mg/kg azithromycin 30 minutes before procedure 20 mg/kg (IV) clindamycin 25 mg/ kg (IM or IV) cefazolin

Heart Failure

Heart failure represents a clinical syndrome that is due to a wide variety of heterogenous etiologies. Heart failure is inability of cardiovascular system to meet the demands of the end organs. Heart failure may result from abnormal contractile function (systolic dysfunction) or impaired relaxation (diastolic dysfunction).

Etiologies

Coronary artery disease (ischemic cardiomyopathy)
- Hypertension
- Cardiomyopathy
- Valvular heart disease
- Pericardial disease
- Incessant tachyarrhythmia
- High output states (thyrotoxicosis, AV fistula, thiamine deficiency).

Symptoms

Dyspnea, orthopnea and paroxysmal nocturnal dyspnea are classic symptoms, but non-specific complaints such as chest discomfort, fatigue, palpitations, dizziness and syncope are not uncommon.

Oral Considerations

For well-compensated patients with heart failures, no special dental modifications are necessary unless the underlying causes for the heart failure require modifications. When patients suffer from uncompensated cardiac heart failure, it is prudent to inquire about the patient's ability to be placed in supine position because lying down flat in a dental chair may cause severe dyspnea in such patients.

Arrhythmia

Abnormalities of cardiac rhythm can be broadly defined as any deviation from the normal cardiac pacemaker and conduction mechanism. Tachyarrhythmias occur as a result of increased automaticity of cardiac pacemaker cells reentry or triggered activity and are defined as any abnormal heart rhythm with a rate > 100 bpm (beats per minute). Bradyarrhythmias occur as a result of sinuatrial node dysfunction and conduction blockade at any level of the conduction tissues including the atrioventricular node, this purkinje system, or distal branches of the left and right bundles. Bradyarrhythmias are associated with heart rates of < 60 bpm. Both tachyarrhythmias and bradyarrhythmias may be hemodynamically well tolerated in patients with normal cardiac function or they may result in cardiovascular collapse if cardiac output is significantly compromised.

Atrial Fibrillation

Atrial fibrillation is a common dysarrhythmia and occurs both with and without structural heart disease. In case of atrial fibrillation, the chaotic atrial activity results in ineffective atrial contraction and in stasis of blood within the left atrium. This stasis may lead to thrombus formation and may increase the risk of embolic events, including cerebral and peripheral embolization. The risk of embolic stroke increases with increasing age, comorbidities and CVD.

The dental protocols for patients with AF included need for antibiotic prophylaxis, the need to alter dental care on the basis of the patient's anticoagulation therapy, and the use of anxiety-reducing strategies.

9

Renal Diseases

CHRONIC RENAL FAILURE

Chronic renal failure can be caused by several diseases that devastate the nephron mass of the kidneys. Some renal considerations affects glomerulus (glomerulonephritis), others involve the renal tubules (polycystic kidney disease); while others interfere with blood perfusion to renal parenchyma (nephrosclerosis).

Etiology of renal disease is diabetes mellitus, hypertension, glomerulonephritis, polycystic kidney disease.

Manifestation of Renal Disease

Two groups of symptoms are present in patients with uremic syndrome: Symptoms related to altered regulatory and excretory functions (fluid volume, electrolyte abnormalities, acid-base imbalance, accumulation of nitrogenous waste and anemia) and a group of clinical symptoms affects the cardiovascular, gastrointestinal, hematologic and other systems.

Biochemical Disturbances

Metabolic acidosis is a common biochemical disturbance experienced by patients with renal disease. As kidney function fails, excretion of hydrogen (H^+) ions diminishes, leading to systemic acidosis that results in lower plasma pH and bicarbonate (HCO_3^-) concentration. Ammonium excretion decreased because of reduced nephron mass, is the most important factor in kidney's ability to eliminate H^+ and regenerate HCO_3^-. These patients often suffer from a moderate acidosis. The symptoms of anorexia, lethargy and nausea frequently observed in patients with uremia may be partly due to this metabolic acidosis.

Gastrointestinal Symptoms

The more common symptoms are nausea, vomiting and anorexia. Gastrointestinal inflammations such as gastritis, duodenitis and esophagitis are common in late renal failure and can affect the entire gastrointestinal tract.

Neurologic Signs and Symptoms

Both central and peripheral nervous systems are involved. As the disease progresses, asterisks and myoclonic jerks may become evident. Central nervous system irritability and eventual seizures may occur. Peripheral neuropathy is commonly present as a result of a disturbance of the conduction mechanism rather than a quantitative loss of nerve fiber. Patient complaints are paresthesia that may progress to eventual muscle weakness, atrophy and finally paralysis. This predominantly affects the lower extremities but can affect upper extremities as well. Rarely facial, oral and paraoral regions can also be affected.

Hematologic Problems

Patients with chronic renal dysfunction will often have hematologic problems, most common anemia and increased bleeding.

Renal Osteodystrophy

Renal osteodystrophy refers to the skeletal changes that result from chronic renal disease and that are caused by disorders in calcium and phosphorus metabolism, abnormal vitamin D metabolism and increased parathyroid activity.

Cardiovascular Manifestations

Hypertension and congestive heart failure are common manifestations of uremic syndrome. The association of circulatory overload and hypertension caused by disturbances in sodium and water balance contributes to an increased prevalence of congestive heart failure.

Respiratory Symptoms

The deep sighing breathing seen in response to metabolic acidosis is seen with uremia. Dyspnea on exertion is a more frequent and often overlooked complaint in patients with progressing disease.

Oral Manifestations

With impaired renal function, a decreased Glomerular Filtration Rate (GFR) and accumulation and retention of various products of renal failure, the oral cavity may show a variety of changes as the body progresses through an azotemic to a uremic state. Some of the presenting signs were an ammonia-like taste and smell, stomatitis, decreased salivary flow, xerostomia and parotitis.

As renal failure develops, one of the early symptoms may be a bad taste and odor in the mouth, particularly in the morning. This uremic factor, an ammoniacal odor, typical of any uremic patient is caused by the high concentration of urea in the saliva and its subsequent breakdown to ammonia. An acute rise in Blood Urea Nitrogen (BUN) level may result in uremic stomatitis, which may appear as an erythemopultaceous form characterized by red mucosa covered with a thick exudates and a pseudomembrane or as an ulcerative form characterized by frank ulcerations with redness and a pultaceous coat. Intraoral changes have been related to BUN level > 150 mg/dl and disappear spontaneously when medical treatment results in lowered BUN level. White plaques called 'uremic frost' occasionally found on the skin can rarely be found intraorally. This uremic frost results from residual urea crystals left on the epithelial surfaces after perspiration evaporates or as a result of decreased salivary flow. A more common oral finding is significant xerostomia probably caused by a combination of direct involvement of salivary glands, chemical inflammation, dehydration, and mouth breathing.

Salivary adenitis can occasionally be seen. Another findings associated with increased salivary urea nitrogen, particularly in children, is a low caries activity. This is observed despite a high sugar intake and poor oral hygiene, suggesting an increased neutralizing capacity of the urea arising from ureal hydrolysis. Other oral manifestations of renal disease are related to renal osteodystrophy (RO). These manifestations usually become evident late in the course of the disease. The classic signs of RO in the mandible and maxilla are bone demineralization, loss of trabeculation, ground-glass appearance, total or partial loss of lamina dura, giant cell lesions or brown tumors and metastatic calcifications. These changes appear most frequently in the mandibular molar region superior to the mandibular canal. The rarefaction in the mandible and maxilla is secondary to generalized osteoporosis. The compact bone of the jaws may become thinned and eventually disappear. This may be evident as loss of the lower border of the mandible, the cortical margins of the inferior dental canal and floor of the antrum and lamina dura. Spontaneous and pathologic fractures may occur with the thinning of these areas of compact bone and may complicate dental extractions.

The radiolucent lesions of hyperparathyroidism are called' Brown tumor' because they contain areas of old hemorrhage and appear brown on clinical inspection. As these tumors increase in size, the resultant expansion may involve the cortex. Although tumor rarely breaks through the periosteum, gingival swelling may occur. The brown tumor lesion contains abundance of multi-nucleated giant cells, fibroblasts, and hemosiderin. This histologic appearance is also consistent with central giant cell tumor and giant cell reparative granuloma. Associated bone changes consist of a generalized osteitis fibrosa, with patches of osteoclastic resorption on all bone surfaces. This is replaced by a vascular connective tissue that represents an abortive formation of coarse-fibered woven bone. This histologic picture also may be seen in fibrous dysplasia, giant cell reparative granuloma, osteomalacia and paget's disease.

Other clinical manifestations of renal osteodystrophy include tooth mobility, malocclusion and metastatic soft tissue calcification. Increasing mobility and drifting of teeth with no apparent pathologic periodontal pocket formation may be seen. Periapical radiolucencies and root resorption may also be associated with this gradual mobility of the dentition. The teeth

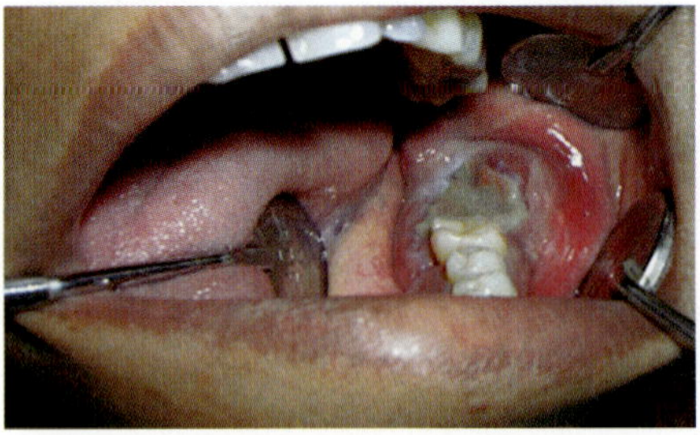

Fig. 9.1: Brown tumor of oral cavity

may be painful to percussion and mastication and positive thermal and electric pulp test responses will be elicited.

Splinting is an useful adjunct to present pain and further drifting, and the splint should be maintained until adequate treatment of the HPTH (hyperparathyroidism) results in bone remineralization. Malocclusion may result from the advanced mobility and drifting of the dentition. Extreme demineralization and collapse of the temporomandibular and paratemporomandibular bones may also produce a malocclusion.

Abnormal bone repair after extraction termed 'socket sclerosis' and radiographically characterized by a lack of lamina dura resorption and by the deposition of sclerotic bone in the confines of the lamina dura, has been reported in patients with renal disease although it is not unique to them.

Enamel hypoplasia is frequently seen in patients whose renal disease started at a young age. The location of the hypoplastic enamel on the permanent teeth corresponds to the age of onset of advanced renal failure. Prolonged corticosteroid therapy may also contribute to this deficiency. Another dental finding is pulpal narrowing and calcifications. In some patients who are on dialysis, severe tooth erosion as a result of the nausea and extensive vomiting that often follows dialysis treatment may be seen. The platelet changes with renal disease itself and with dialysis therapy, gingival bleeding may be a common patient complaint.

Oral consideration: Management of the patient with renal disease

- Before treatment
  - Determine dialysis schedule and treat on day after dialysis.
  - Consult with patient's nephrologist for recent laboratory tests and discussion of antibiotic prophylaxis
  - Identify arm with vascular access and type; avoid taking blood pressure measurement/injection of medication on this arm.
  - Evaluate patient for hypertension/hypotension.
  - Obtain routine annual dental radiographs to establish presence and follow manifestation of renal osteodystrophy.
  - Consider antibiotic prophylaxis when appropriate.

- During treatment
  - Perform a thorough history and physical examination for presence of oral manifestations.
  - Use adjunctive hemostatic acids during oral/periodontal surgical procedures.
  - Maintain patient in a comfortable uncramped position in the dental chair.
  - Allow patient to walk or stand intermittently during long procedures.
- After treatment
  - Use postsurgical hemostatic agents
  - Institute therapy for xerostomia when appropriate
  - Consider use of postoperative antibiotics for traumatic procedures.
  - Adjust dosages of postoperative medications according to extent of renal failure.

Drugs to limit or avoid when treating dialysis patients:

Magnesium content	–	Antacids (milk of magnesia), laxatives
Potassium content	–	IV fluids Salt substitutes Massive penicillin therapy
Sodium content	–	Carbenicillin IV fluid
Acidifying effects	–	Ascorbic acid Ammonium chloride Non-steroidal anti-inflammatory agents
Catabolic effects	–	Tetracyclines Steroids
Nephro toxicity	–	Phenacetin Ketorolac Cephalosporins (long term especially combined with gentamicin)
Alkalosis	–	Absorbed antacids Carbenicillin (large doses) Penicillin (large doses)

LIVER DISEASES

The liver consists of hepatocytes which are organized for optimal contact with sinusoids (leading to and from blood vessels) and bile ducts. The functions of liver are mainly the metabolism, breakdown and excretion of drugs and endogenous products such as ammonia, bilirubin and sex steroids. Most drugs are metabolized in the liver. In the liver, drugs may undergo first-pass metabolism, in which they are activated or inactivated before they enter the systemic circulation. Ammonia is converted to urea, which is excreted into the urine by the kidneys. Many important substances such as albumin, blood clotting factors, transporter proteins, complement, cholesterol, and bile components are produced. The liver produces most of the coagulation factors apart from the anti-hemophilic factors. The liver stores substances such as glycogen, fat soluble vitamins, folate, vitamin B_{12} and minerals such as copper and iron. The liver helps to maintain body homeostasis by regulation of blood levels of substances such as cholesterol and glucose.

VIRAL HEPATITIS

Hepatitis is a term for liver inflammation and it can result from many insults, including infections, drugs and poisons. The term viral hepatitis refers to infection by hepatitis B, D and C viruses.

Hepatitis B

It is caused by the hepatitis B virus and is a serious disease. It can cause life long infection, cirrhosis of liver, liver cancer, liver failure and death. Spread of hepatitis is mainly by blood or blood products.

Clinical Features

The HBV infection ranges from subclinical infections without jaundice to fulminating hepatitis, acute hepatic failure and death. The prodromal period of 1–2 weeks is characterized by anorexia, malaise and nausea. Hepatitis viremia precedes the clinical illness by weeks or months and lasts for some weeks before clearing completely. As jaundice becomes clinically evident, the stools become pale and urine dark due to bilirubinuria. The liver is enlarged and tender and pruritus may be troublesome. Muscle pain, arthralgia and rashes are more common in hepatitis B. Complications of hepatitis B include a carrier state, chronic state, chronic infection, cirrhosis, liver cancer or death.

Oral Considerations

The following drugs are contraindicated,

- Analgesics such as aspirin, codeine, indomethacin, mefenamic acid, opioids, paracetamol/acetaminophen .
- Antimicrobials such as aminoglycosides, azithromycin, azole antifungals, clarithromycin, clindamycin, coamoxiclov, cotrimoxazole, doxycycline, erythromycin estolate, metronidazole, roxithromycin, talampicillin.
- Local anesthetics – lidocaine.
- Corticosteroids – Prednisone

Patients with normal platelet counts and normal prothrombin time can undergo dental intervention safely. Bleeding tendencies may be there if platelet count is low or prothrombin time is prolonged. Pure parotid saliva does not contain HbsAg, but saliva collected from oral cavity may contain HBV (from serum through gingival exudate) and may be source for non-parental transmission. Hepatitis can be transmitted by human bites. Blood, plasma or serum can be infectious. As little as 0.0000001 ml of HBsAg positive serum can transmit hepatitis B.

Hepatitis C

Hepatitis C virus infection accounts worldwide for at least 90% of post-transfusion non-A non-B hepatitis. HCV is also responsible for much sporadic viral hepatitis, particularly in intravenous drug abusers.

Clinical Features

Hepatitis C has similar incubation period to hepatitis B, usually less than 60 but up to 150 days. Eighty to ninety percent of infected persons have no signs and symptoms. Clinical hepatitis C has less severe and shorter illness than hepatitis B. A greater proportion of patients infected with HCV have abnormal liver function tests after one year and may go to chronic liver disease and some develop liver cancer or die. Hepatitis C virus is

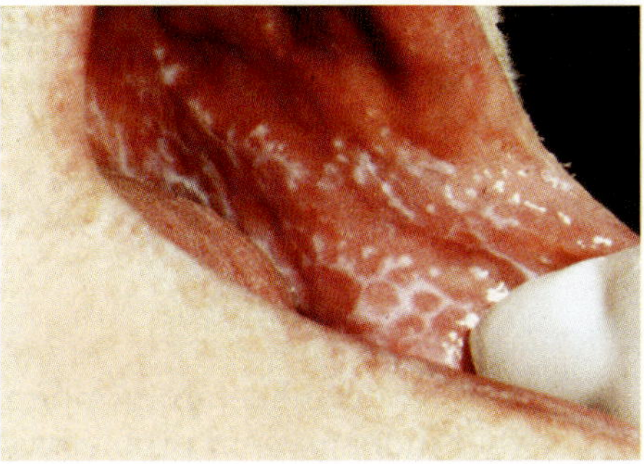

Fig. 9.2: Lichen planus

associated in some population with sicca syndrome, lichen planus, lymphoma, cryoglobulinemia and other extrahepatic manifestations.

Oral Considerations

Hepatitis C virus has been found in saliva and infection had followed human bite. HCV may be associated with oral features such as sicca syndrome, non-Hodgkin's lymphoma and with lichen planus.

Chronic Hepatitis

Chronic hepatitis is the term for hepatitis which persists longer than 6 months and includes a spectrum of disorders between acute hepatitis and cirrhosis.

Etiology

The most important causes of chronic hepatitis are HCV accounting 60 to 70% of cases and up to 50% of cirrhosis, end-stage liver disease and liver cancer; idiopathic, with prominent immune features.

Clinical Features

About 70% cases develop insidiously but some follow acute hepatitis. Many patients are asymptomatic and the disorders remain subclinical for years or decades. Malaise, anorexia and fatique are common, sometimes with low grade fever and upper abdominal discomfort. Signs of chronic liver disease that may develop include splenomegaly, spider naevi, ascites and fluid retention, but jaundice is variable and often absent. In autoimmune hepatitis, multisystem manifestations are common, especially in young women and include acne, arthralgia, amenorrhea, hemolytic anemia, nephritis, pulmonary fibrosis, thyroiditis and ulcerative colitis.

Oral Considerations

Hepatotoxic agents, aspirin and acetaminophen/paracetamol should be avoided. Other management problems such as chronic liver disease, HBV or HCV carriage, corticosteroids, complicating disorders such as diabetes, Wilson's disease are included. Sjögren's syndrome is relatively common and oral lichenoid lesions may develop.

Cirrhosis

In cirrhosis of liver, there is liver cell necrosis and inflammation followed by fibrosis, nodular regeneration and vascular derangement. Liver function deteriorates and flow of blood through the organs becomes obstructed. It is a non-specific reaction causing liver damage, but most is idiopathic. Cirrhosis is a common sequelae to hepatitis C virus or alcohol related damage. Alcohol injures the liver by blocking the normal metabolism of protein, fats and carbohydrates. Cirrhosis develops after more than a decade of heavy drinking but the amount of alcohol that can injure the liver varies greatly from person to person. Non-alcoholic steotohepatitis in which fat builds up in the liver and causes scar tissue, is associated with diabetes, protein, malnutrition, obesity, coronary artery disease or corticosteroid treatment.

Clinical Features

Cirrhosis affects the middle-aged or elderly and is asymptomatic in its earlier stages. Anorexia, malaise and weight loss are common. Jaundice, splenomegaly, ascites, gastrointestinal hemorrhage, palmar erythema, spider naevi, finger clubbing, opaque nails, pigmentation, fluid retention, bruising, gynaecomastia, testicular atrophy and other features may be present. Alcoholic cirrhosis may have parotid swelling, pancreatitis or gastric ulceration. It is a lethal disorder and result in serious complications from hepatocellular damage or portal venous hypertension and includes haematemesis (vomiting of blood) which can cause anemia and death. Thrombocytopenia from splenomegaly and low blood clotting factor levels leading to bleeding tendency that worsen the hemorrhage from esophageal varices. Most infections are with normal gut aerobic bacteria or gram positive bacteria, invasive dental or oral surgical procedures may increase the risk and since the mortality approaches 30%, antibiotic prophylaxis must be considered. Other complications are diabetes mellitus, peptic ulceration, renal dysfunction and hepatoma.

Oral Considerations

The physician should be contacted if surgery, general anesthesia or drug therapy are needed. Surgery is hazardous, particularly in view of bleeding tendencies and also because of diabetes, anemia, drug therapy, HCV or HBV carriage, poor wound healing and a liability to peritonitis. Spontaneous bacterial peritonitis is a potential problem in cirrhosis with ascites. Invasive dental or oral surgical procedures may increase the risk and mortality approaches 30%, antibiotic prophylaxis may be considered. Amoxycillin orally 2–3 gm with metronidazole 1 hour preoperatively or intravenous imipenem are recommended. There is association between liver cirrhosis and oral carcinoma.

LIVER CANCER

Cancer of hepatocytes is also termed hepatocellular carcinoma or malignant hepatoma. Metastatic cancer to liver from colon, lungs, breasts, uterus, or other parts of the body is more common. The risk factors for hepatocellular carcinoma include male gender, old age, positive family history, chronic HBV or HCV, cirrhosis, aflatoxin-a mould which forms on peanuts, corn, and other nuts and grains and long term oral contraceptive use.

Clinical Features

Early cases cause no symptoms. Later manifestations may include wasting, jaundice, pain in the right upper abdomen, swelling, loss of appetite, weakness, nausea and vomiting and fever.

Oral Considerations

No significant dental considerations other than those applying to other causes of severe liver disease.

Extrahepatic Biliary Obstruction

The causes for biliary obstruction are mainly gall stones and carcinoma of the pancreas. Gallstones are common with advancing age, particularly in females. 10 to 20% of adults have gall stones, but most are symptomless.

Clinical Features

Gall stones are asymptomatic. However, passage of stones into the bile ducts can cause severe pain due to biliary colic, acute cholecystitis or acute pancreatitis. Extrahepatic biliary obstruction causes jaundice, pruritis, dark urine and pale stools. Biliary obstruction can lead to impaired absorption of fats and vitamin K.

Oral Considerations

Excessive bleeding results from vitamin K malabsorption. Surgical intervention should be deferred in the presence of jaundice until hemostatic function returns to normal. If surgery is to be performed essentially vitamin K_1 is to be given parenterally at a dose of 10 mg daily for several days. General anesthesia in jaundiced patient may lead to renal failure (hepatorenal syndrome).

10 Hematological Diseases

ANEMIA

Anemia is decrease in number of red blood cells, hemoglobin or both. The reduction in hemoglobin may result from blood loss, as in common iron deficiency anemia, from increased destruction of red blood cells as in hemolytic anemias, from decreased production of red cells, as in pernicious anemias and folic acid deficiency anemias or from combinations of these three.

General symptoms of all anemias include pallor of skin, palpebral conjunctiva and nail beds, dyspnea and easy fatigability.

Iron deficiency anemia may result from chronic blood loss such as menopausal bleeding, bleeding hemorrhoids or a bleeding malignant lesion or ulcer in the gastrointestinal tract.

Oral Manifestations

The major oral sign of iron deficiency anemia is pallor of the mucosa. In addition, the oral epithelial cells become atrophic, with loss of normal keratinization. The tongue may become smooth due to atrophy of the filiform and fungi form papillae and glossodynia can be a presenting or associated symptoms. In long standing cases esophageal strictures or webs can develop, resulting in dysphagia.

Oral Considerations

Dental patients presenting with symptoms of anemia or oral signs suggestive of this condition should have a complete blood count (CBC) with differential. Elective oral surgical or periodontal procedures should not be performed on patients with marked anemia because of the potential for increased bleeding and impaired wound healing. When hemoglobin levels fall below 10 g/dl, the low oxygen tension affects the rheologic interactions between the cellular components of blood, mainly platelets and endothelium, decreasing their ability to clot effectively. General anesthesia should not be administered unless the hemoglobin is atleast 10 g/dl.

Anemia Owing to Hemolysis

The hemolytic anemia results from decreased survival of erythrocytes, either episodically or continuously.

Hemolytic anemia may be caused by overwhelming infections and toxins, cardiac valvular prostheses, chronic liver disease and transfusion reactions. Certain intracorpuscular causes also result in hemolytic anemia.

Oral Manifestations

When sufficient hemolysis has taken place to produce anemia, pallor results. This is most easily observed in the nail beds and palpebral conjunctiva. Pallor of oral mucosa, evident in the soft palate, tongue, and sublingual tissues, is also observable as the anemia progresses. Hemolytic anemia produces jaundice caused by the hyperbilirubenemia secondary to erythrocyte destruction. This is best seen in the sclera, but the skin, soft palate and tissues of the floor of the mouth also become icteric as the serum bilirubin increases.

Oral Consideration

The severity of anemia and its correction should be evaluated before major dental interventions because the decline in hemoglobin can reach 3 to 4 g/dl during hemolytic episodes. Blood transfusion may be used prior to dental treatment in severe cases. The erythroid elements of bone marrow are hyperplastic in an attempt to compensate for the anemia. This hyperplasia produces a characteristic appearance on the dental radiograph. Because of the enlargement of medullary spaces, the trabeculae become prominent, creating increased bone radiolucency with prominent lamellar striations.

Drugs that might induce hemolysis such as dapsone, sulfasalazine, and phenacetin should be avoided. The hemolytic episodes are self limited and most patients with drug or infection-induced hemolysis recover fully following treatment.

LEUKEMIA

Leukemia is a malignancy affecting the WBC's of the bone marrow. This neoplastic process is characterized by differentiation and proliferation of malignantly transformed hematopoietic stem cell, leading to suppression of normal cells.

Acute Leukemia

The acute leukemias are malignancies of hematopoietic progenitor cells, which consequently fail to mature and differentiate. They are divided into two major groups—acute lymphocytic leukemia (ALL) and acute myelogenous leukemia (AML).

In older patients, AML may be preceded by a preleukemic or myelodysplastic syndrome, with generalized bone marrow abnormalities affecting RBCs, leukocytes and platelets. Leukemia preceded by these syndromes responds poorly to therapy.

Clinical Manifestations

Acute leukemia occurs at any age, but ALL is commonly found in children, whereas AML occurs more frequently in adults. The symptoms and signs of acute leukemia result from either bone marrow suppression or infiltration of leukemic cells into other organs and tissues. The bone marrow changes cause anemia, thrombocytopenia, and a decrease in normally functioning neutrophils. The anemia results in pallor, shortness of breath and fatigue, which is the most common presenting symptom.

Thrombocytopenia causes spontaneous bleeding such as petechiae, ecchymoses, epistaxis, melena, gingival bleeding when platelet count falls below 25,000/mm^3.

Although leukemic patients often present with a greatly increased number of leukocytes, these leukemic cells do not function normally, resulting in defective migration, phagocytosis or bactericidal action. Infection is therefore a frequent complication of the disease and is the most common cause of morbidity and mortality. Fever is an early sign of disease owing to recurrent infections of the lungs, urinary tract, skin, most rectum and upper respiratory tract. Localized tumors consisting of leukemic cells are called 'choloromas'.

Chronic Leukemia

Chronic leukemias are characterized by the presence of a large number of well-differentiated cells in the bone marrow, peripheral blood and tissues and a prolonged clinical course even without therapy. This distinguishes chronic leukemia from acute leukemia in which immature cells predominate, and the untreated clinical course leads to death in months. The two major types are chronic myelocytic leukemia (CML) and chronic lymphocytic leukemia (CLL).

Chronic Myelocytic Leukemia

CML occurs most frequently in patients between the ages of 30 and 50 years. No symptoms are noted by the patient during the first few years, and the disease may be discovered during a routine examination when splenomegaly or an elevated WBC is noted. Early signs and symptoms are usually secondary to anemia or the packing of leukocytes into the spleen and bone marrow. The anemia causes weakness, fatigue, and dyspnea on exertion. As the disease progresses thrombocytopenia can cause petechiae, ecchymoses and hemorrhage.

Chronic Lymphocytic Leukemia

CLL results from a slowly progressing malignancy involving the lymphocytes. CLL occurs most frequently in males older than 40 years, with 60 years being the most common age of onset. As a result of slow natural history, it is not uncommon for the disease to be detected incidentally by routine hematology before any signs or symptoms is apparent. The asymptomatic phase of the disease may last for years, but eventually signs and symptoms of infiltration of leukemic cells in the bone marrow, lymph nodes or other tissues appear. Bone marrow infiltration causes anemia and thrombocytopenia, resulting in pallor, weakness, dyspnea and purpura, infiltration of other tissues causes lymphadenopathy, splenomegaly, hepatomegaly and leukemic infiltrates of skin or mucosa. Cervical lymphadenopathy and tonsillar enlargement are frequent head and neck signs of CLL.

Patients with CLL exhibit some degree of hypogammaglobulinemia with an increased susceptibility to bacterial infection. Infection with varicella-zoster virus also is common.

Late in the disease, massive lymphadenopathy may cause intestinal or urethral obstruction and obstructive jaundice.

Oral and Dental Consideration

Oral complications are common throughout the clinical course of the disease, dental management is complex, and the mouth is a potential source of morbidity and mortality. Oral signs and symptoms are common; the dentist may be the first clinician to suspect the disease. Head and neck signs result from leukemic infiltrates or marrow failure. These include cervical lymphadenopathy, oral bleeding, gingival infiltrates, infections and oral ulcers. Thromobocytopenia and anemia caused by marrow suppression from disease and chemotherapy result in pallor of the mucosa, petechiae and ecchymoses, as well as gingival bleeding. Spontaneous gingival bleeding is common when the platelet count falls below 20,000/mm^3. Topical treatment to stop gingival bleeding should always include removal of obvious local irritants and direct pressure, use of absorbable gelatin or collagen sponges, topical thrombin or the placement of microfibrillar collagen held in place by packing or splints (Fig. 10.1).

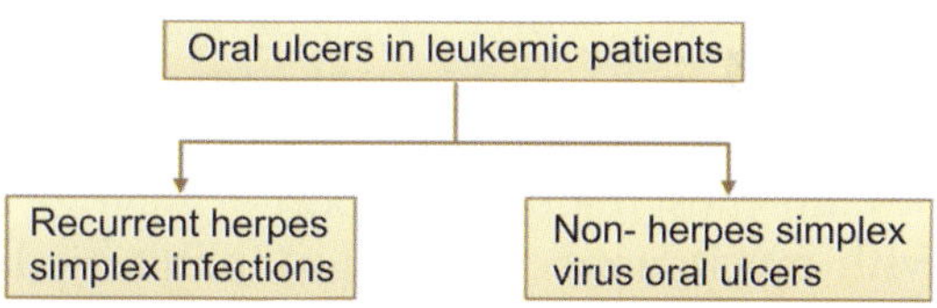

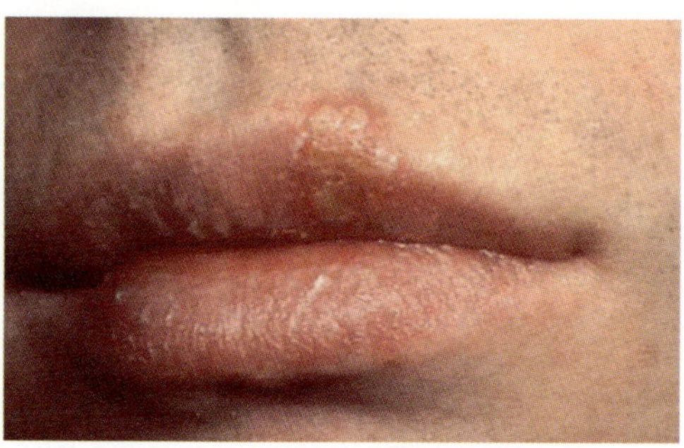

Fig. 10.1: Herpes simplex infection

Oral Ulcers

Oral mucosal ulcers are common findings in leukemic patients taking chemotherapy and are frequently caused by the direct effect of chemotherapeutic drugs on the oral mucosal cells. The ulcers are characteristically large, irregular and foul smelling and are surrounded by pale mucosa caused by anemia and a lack of normal inflammatory response.

Oral Infections

Oral infection is a serious potentially fatal complication in neutropenic leukemic patients. Candidiasis is a common oral fungal infection, but infections with other fungi such as Histoplasma, Aspergillus or Phycomycetes, fungi also may begin on the oral tissues. When these lesions are suspected, a biopsy specimen, a fine needle aspiration, or a cytology smear must be obtained because a culture alone is not a reliable test for these organisms.

Diagnosis of dental infections, particularly periodontal and pericoronal infections, is difficult in neutropenic leukemic patients because normal inflammation is absent. The early diagnosis of oral infection is imperative because it has been demonstrated that oral flora is a significant source of potentially life-threatening infections with gram-positive and gram-negative bacilli.

Oral signs also may result from the presence of leukemic infiltrates. These are most frequently reported as gingival infiltrates in patients with myelomonocytic and monoblastic leukemia or acute promyelocytic leukemia. Leukemia infiltrates involving palate, alveolar bone, and dental pulp also have been reported, leukemic infiltrates may cause oral signs and symptoms because of the involvement of the fifth and seventh cranial nerves.

Lymphoma

The lymphomas are a group of malignant solid tumors involving cells of lymphoreticular or immune system, such as B-lymphocytes, T-lymphocytes and monocytes. The etiology is unknown but risks factors include immunodeficiency states, viral infections, and chemical exposure. The initial tumor formation in lymphoma is in the secondary lymphatic tissues, where normal tissue is replaced by malignant lymphocytes.

Lymphomas are divided into two major categories—Hodgkin's disease and non-Hodgkin's lymphoma. These diseases usually begin in the lymph nodes, but may be the first diagnosed in extranodal lymphoid tissue.

Hodgkin's Disease

Hodgkin's disease is a malignant lymphatic disease. The etiology remains unknown but it is probably culmination of diverse pathologic processes such as viral infections, environmental exposures, and genetically determined host response.

Males have an increased incidence of Hodgkin's disease and the disease has two peaks of highest incidence. The first peak occurs during the second and third decades of life, and the second peak occurs after the fifth decade.

Clinical Manifestations

The most common presentation of Hodgkin's disease is a painless enlargement of lymph nodes in a patient without other symptoms of disease. The cervical lymph nodes are the initial sites of detection in more than 50% of cases. Early involvement of the axillary, inguinal and mediastinal nodes is also common, fever, weight loss, pruritus or night sweats are other symptoms. The involved peripheral nodes are non-tender and feel rubbery. The presentation of asymptomatic enlarged lymph nodes is most common in younger patients with Hodgkin's disease and is consistent with histologic classification of lymphocyte predominance or nodular sclerosis. In older patients with increased risk of developing the lymphocyte depleted or mixed cellularity histologic patter, systemic symptoms such as malaise, fever and night sweats, may precede noticeable lymphadenopathy.

As the disease progresses, signs and symptoms arise from pressure and obstruction caused enlarging nodes. Further progression of disease leads to invasion of bone marrow, lungs, liver, bones and spinal cord. When the disease is generalized, the immunodeficiency leads to increased susceptibility to viral and fungal infections.

Non-Hodgkin's Lymphoma

The group of malignant disorders known as non-Hodgkin's lymphoma arises from B or T lymphocytes.

Clinical Manifestations

The most common presentation of non-Hodgkin's lymphoma is a painless persistent enlargement of the lymph nodes, but extranodal lesions occur more commonly than in Hodgkin's lymphoma, especially in the intermediate and high-grade forms of the disease. Non-Hodgkin's lymphoma may be detected in Waldeyer's ring, gastrointestinal tract, the spleen, skin and bone marrow. Non-Hodgkin's lymphoma is more common in patients older than 40 years, signs and symptoms depend on the site of involvement and result from the pressure of enlarged lymph nodes or infiltration.

Oral Considerations

Asymptomatic enlargement of the cervical lymph node chains is common early sign of lymphoma, and the dentist plays a significant role in early detection by routine examination of the neck. Suspicion of lymphoma should increase when lymphadenopathy appears without signs of infection, more than one lymph node chain is involved or a lymph node of 1 cm or greater in diameter persists for more than 1 month.

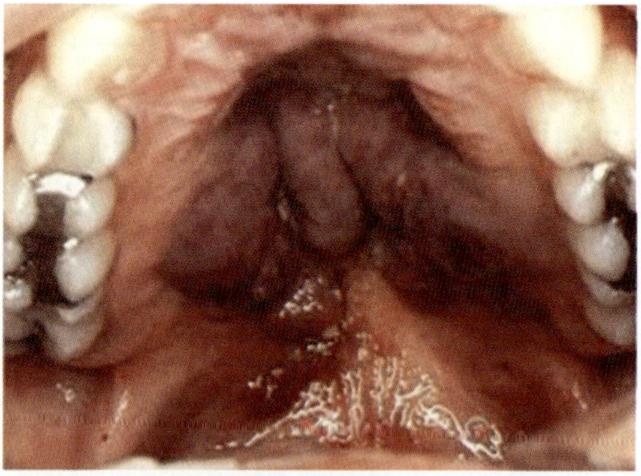

Fig. 10.2: Non-Hodgkin's lymphoma

Non-Hodgkin's lymphoma is more frequent in immune comprised patients, including patients with AIDS and those receiving immunosuppressive drug therapies. The palatal lesion has been described as slow-growing, painless, bluish, soft masses and they have been confused with minor salivary gland tumors. Oral non-Hodgkin's lymphoma presents as a gingival mass, tongue mass or intraosseous lesion. Isolated loose teeth, paresthesia of the face and major salivary gland enlargement may also be presenting signs of non-Hodgkin's lymphoma.

When lymphoma is included in differential diagnosis of an oral lesion, a biopsy specimen which has not been traumatized should be taken from the center of the lesion and sent to an experienced pathologist. The pathologist should be informed of the possibility of lymphoma because non-Hodgkin's lymphoma is easily confused with benign lymphoproliferative disorders. Special staining with Giemsa and periodic acid-schiff and typing with immunohistochemistry are helpful in making the diagnosis of non-Hodgkin's lymphoma.

MULTIPLE MYELOMA

Multiple myeloma is a malignant neoplasm of plasma cells that is characterized by the production of pathologic M proteins, bone lesions, kidney disease, hyperviscosity and hypercalcemia. It occurs most often in patients older than 50 years of age.

Skeletal pain is the most common presenting symptom and is caused by bone lysis that may result either directly from accumulation of tumor cells or indirectly from osteoclast-activating factors secreted by the malignant myeloma cells. Approximately 80% of patients with multiple myeloma have bone lesions and pathologic fractures are frequent complication. The most common radiographic abnormality is the presence of "punched-out" radiolucent lesions (plasmacytomas), but generalized osteoporosis may occur in the absence of these discrete punched-out lesions.

Renal failure is also common complications resulting from a combination of amyloidosis, hypercalcemia and infiltration of malignant cells. Amyloid may also deposit in the heart, liver, nervous system or other organs, interfering with normal function. Deposition of this amorphous protein under the skin or mucosa is also common. Diagnosis is based on serum M-proteins demonstrated with serum protein electrophoresis or immunoelectrophoresis or on Bence Jones proteins, which are monoclonal immunoglobulin light chains detected in 24 hours urine specimens. Bone marrow biopsy results reveal atypical plasma cells.

Oral Manifestations

Approximately 5 to 30% of myeloma patients have jaw lesions, and accidental discovery of lesions in the jaws may be the first evidence of this disease. Patient may experience pain, swelling numbness of the jaws, and unexplained mobility of the teeth. Mandible is more frequently involved in multiple myeloma. Extraosseous lesions also occur in a significant number of patients although a majority of lesions are asymptomatic.

Oral amyloidosis occurs as complication of this disease. Clinically tongue may be enlarged and studded with small garnet colored enlargements, including nodes on the cheeks and lips. Special staining with Congo red can be used. Biopsy specimen to detect amyloidosis must include muscle tissue from the mucobuccal fold or tongue (Fig. 10.3).

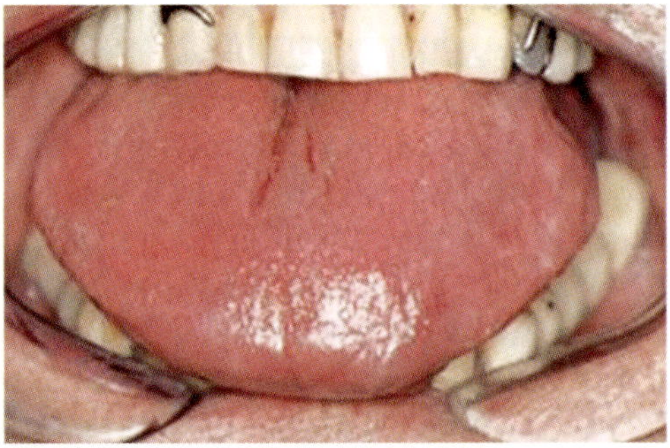

Fig. 10.3: Amyloidosis of tongue

Oral Considerations

Hemorrhage and infection are the dentist's major concerns when treating a patient with multiple myeloma. Bleeding may result from several causes, including thrombocytopenia abnormal platelet function, abnormal coagulation, or hyperviscosity. If surgery is necessary results of platelet count, bleeding time, prothrombin time and partial thromboplastin time should be obtained. If hyperviscosity is present, excess bleeding may occur even if these tests are normal and a hematology consultation should be considered.

The dentist should determine whether the patient has an increased susceptibility to bacterial infection due to hypergammaglobulinemia, bone marrow failure or complications of cancer chemotherapy.

11 Immunologic Diseases

SCLERODERMA

Scleroderma is a multisystem connective tissue disease that involves hardening of the skin and mucosa, smooth-muscle atrophy and fibrosis of internal organs. This disease has higher age-specific incidence rate.

Subtypes – Localized scleroderma
– Progressive systemic sclerosis

Localized Scleroderma

Localized scleroderma refers to scleroderma primarily involving the skin, with minimal systemic features. Three major types of localized scleroderma exist; morphea, generalized morphea and linear scleroderma. Morphea begins with no laceous skin patches that enlarge, become indurated, and eventually lose hair and the ability to sweat. Later in the course of the disease, the lesion 'burn out' and appears as a hypo- or hyper-pigmented area depressed below the level of the skin. A smaller number of patients develop numerous larger lesions that coalesce and these patients are said to have generalized morphea. Patients with either type of morphea usually have a benign course characterized by softening of the lesions over time. Linear scleroderma is a form of the localized disease that may develop during childhood.

Progressive Systemic Sclerosis

Progressive systemic sclerosis is a multisystem disease characterized by the inflammation and fibrosis of many organs. It occurs four times more frequently in female with its highest incidence occurring between the ages of 25 and 50 years. There are two major subsets: Limited cutaneous scleroderma and diffuse cutaneous scleroderma. Patients with limited scleroderma often have a long history of Raynaud's phenomenon before the appearance of other symptoms.

Diffuse scleroderma patients have a more acute onset, with constitutional symptoms, arthritis, carpal tunnel syndrome and marked swelling of the hands and legs.

Clinical Manifestation

Progressive systemic sclerosis is a chronic multisystem disorder characterized by intense fibrosis involving skin, vasculature, synovium, skeletal muscles, and internal organs.

Raynaud's Phenomenon

Raynaud's phenomenon, a paroxysmal vasospasm of the fingers that results in a change in the color of the fingertips as a response to cold or emotion, is the most common findings of progressive systemic sclerosis.

Cutaneous Manifestations

The thickening of the skin of progressive systemic sclerosis patients always begins in the fingers. Early skin changes, starting with pitting edema, often involve the whole hand and the extremities. In several months, the edema is replaced by a tightening and hardening of the skin, which results in difficulty in moving the affected parts.

Musculoskeletal Manifestations

Polyarthralgias and morning stiffness affecting both small and large joints are frequent in patients with scleroderma. Inflammatory joint pain with markedly swollen fingers often appears to be true synovitis and can lead to the premature diagnosis of rheumatoid arthritis.

Gastrointestinal Manifestations

Distal esophageal motor dysfunction is the most frequent gastrointestinal finding; it results from weakness and incoordination of esophageal heart failure. Patchy replacement of the myocardium and the conduction system by fibrous tissue occurs in most patients.

Pulmonary Manifestations

Pulmonary interstitial fibrosis is now the most frequent cause of death in patients with scleroderma since renal disease has become a treatable complication. Patients with either limited or diffuse scleroderma can develop interstitial disease although it tends to be more severe in patients with diffuse scleroderma.

Renal Manifestations

Renal involvement was the most dreaded and deadly complication of scleroderma. Renal crisis is characterized by malignant hypertension, which can rapidly progress to renal failure.

Oral Manifestations

- The lips become rigid and the oral aperture narrows considerably.
- Skin folds are lost around the mouth, giving a mask-like appearance to the face.
- Tongue can also become hard and rigid, making speaking and swallowing difficult.
- Involvement of oesophagus causes dysphagia.
- Oral telangiectasia is equally prevalent in both limited and diffuse forms and is most commonly observed on the hard palate and lips.

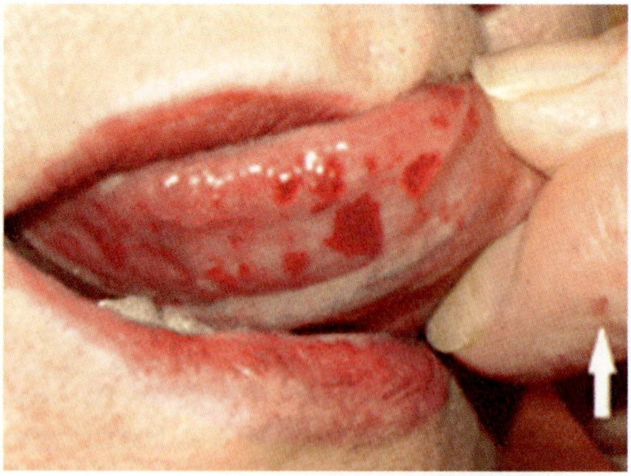

Fig. 11.1: Oral telangiectasia

- When the soft tissues around the temporomandibular joint are affected, they restrict movement of the mandible causing pseudoankylosis.
- The linear form of localized scleroderma may involve the face as well as underlying bone and teeth.

Dental radiographs include uniform thickening of periodontal ligament in less than 10 % of patients. Other characteristic radiographic findings include calcinosis of the soft tissues around the jaws. When facial tissues and muscles of mastication are extensively involved, the pressure exerted will cause resorption of the mandible. This resorption is particularly apparent at the angle of the mandible at the attachment of the masseter muscle. The coronoid process, condyle, or area of attachment of the diagastric muscles may also be damaged by continual pressure.

Patients may also have oral disease secondary to drug therapy or xerostomia. Gingival hyperplasia can result from the use of calcium channel blockers. Pemphigus, blood dyscrasias or lichenoid reaction may result from penicillamine use. Xerostomia results in an increased susceptibility to dental caries, candida infections and periodontal disease.

Oral Considerations

Physical limitation is most common problem in the dental treatment which is caused by narrowing of the oral aperture and rigidity of the tongue. The oral opening may be increased an average of 5 mm stretching exercises. One particularly effective technique is the use of an increasing number of tongue blades between the posterior teeth to stretch the facial tissues. Mechanical devices that assist the patient in performing the stretching exercises are available. If these approaches are insufficient, a bilateral commissurotomy may be necessary.

The extent of heart, lung or kidney involvement should be considered while treating patients with diffuse scleroderma.

Patients with extensive resorption of the angle of mandible are at risk for developing pathologic fractures from minor trauma, including dental extractions.

RHEUMATOID ARTHRITIS

Rheumatoid arthritis (RA) is a disease characterized by inflammation of the synovial membrane. While degenerative joint disease (osteoarthritis), which is localized to the joints in middle-aged and elderly individuals, rheumatoid arthritis affects people of all age groups and affects other organs including muscles and hematopoietic system. Pathogenesis of rheumatoid arthritis is unknown but it appears to be multifactorial involving genetic, immune, and infectious etiologies.

Clinical Manifestations

The initial symptom in majority of patients with rheumatoid arthritis is non-specific weakness and fatigue, which may precede joint symptoms by several months. This is followed by symmetric polyarthritis characterized by a complaint of stiffness and spindle shaped swelling of the involved joints. The proximal interphalangeal joints of the fingers and metacarpophalangeal joints of the hands are most commonly involved; the wrists, elbows, knees and ankles also are frequently involved, including the temporomandibular joint and the cricoarytenoid joint of the larynx. The joints that are affected with rheumatoid arthritis become red, swollen and warm to touch. Muscle atrophy around the affected joint is common.

Extracapsular manifestations include subcutaneous nodules (especially overpressure points), enlargement of the lymph nodes and spleen, chronic skin ulcers from a diffuse arthritis, pleural effusion, and pulmonary fibrosis. Rheumatoid granulomas may affect the heart, the eyes or the brain.

Oral Signs

The treatment of rheumatoid arthritis can cause oral manifestations. The long-term use of methotrexate and other antirheumatic agents such as D-penicillamine and NSAIDs can cause stomatitis. Cyclosporine may cause gingival overgrowth. Patients with long-standing active rheumatoid arthritis have an increased incidence of periodontal disease, including loss of alveolar bone and teeth.

Oral Considerations

The most common complications that affect dental treatment relates to the toxicity of the drugs used to treat rheumatoid arthritis. The most common adverse effects of NSAIDs involve the gastrointestinal tract and the kidneys. In addition, many patients take aspirin at dosages approaching 5 gm per day or take an equivalent dosage of NSAIDs. These drugs affect platelet function, causing a prolongation of the bleeding time and possible hemorrhage after surgery.

Patients with severe rheumatoid arthritis who have had joints surgically replaced with prosthetic joints may require prophylactic antibiotic therapy before invasive dental procedure.

Antibiotic prophylaxis should be considered for patients who will be undergoing dental procedure that are associated with a higher incidence of bacteremia. Such procedures include dental extractions, periodontal surgery, implant placement, replacement of avulsed teeth, endodontic therapy beyond the apex, intraligamentary local anesthetic injections, placement of orthodontic bands and any procedure in which bleeding is anticipated.

Patients with Sjögren's syndrome may require additional instructions in personal oral care, instructions on diet and dietary modifications, home clinical fluoride therapy treatment for xerostomia, more frequent recall visits and radiography and more conservative treatment plans.

12

Infectious Diseases

Certain bacteria, viruses and fungi produce diseases which are manifested in or about the oral cavity. Some of these diseases or lesions are of a specific nature and are produced by a specific microorganism. This microbial specificity or non-specificity is characteristic of infectious diseases wherever they may occur in the body and is necessarily confined to those of the oral cavity.

BACTERIAL INFECTIONS

Tuberculosis

Tuberculosis is a specific infectious granulomatous disease caused by *Mycobacterium tuberculosis*. It commonly affects lungs but also affects the intestines, meninges, bones, joints, lymph glands, skin and other tissues of the body.

The interaction of the bacilli and the host begins when droplet nuclei from infectious patients are inhaled. The majority of the bacilli are trapped and exhaled by ciliary action and a fraction less than 10% enters alveoli. Initial stages are asymptomatic and about 2 or 4 weeks after infection tissue damaging and macrophage activating responses develop. With development of specific immunity and accumulation of a large number of activated macrophages at the site of primary lesion, granulomatous or tubercles are formed. The hard tubercle consists of epithelioid cells, Langhans giant cells, plasma cells and fibroblasts. These lesions develop when host resistance is high.

Clinical Features

The general clinical signs and symptoms of tuberculosis are often remarkably inconspicuous. The patient may suffer episodic fever and chills, but easy fatigability and malaise are often the chief early features of the disease. There may be gradual loss of weight accompanied by a persistent cough with or without associated hemoptysis.

Tuberculosis is either pulmonary or extrapulmonary. Extrapulmonary sites include lymph nodes, pleura, genitourinary tract, bones, joints, meninges and peritoneum. As a result of hematogenous dissemination in HIV infected individuals, the extrapulmonary type is seen more commonly.

Primary pulmonary TB is seen in children, symptoms of post-primary TB or secondary TB include fever, cough, chest pain and hemoptysis. Tuberculosis infection of submandibular and cervical lymph nodes or scrofula, a tuberculous lymphadenitis may progress to the formation of an actual abscess or remain as a typical granulomatous lesion. In either case, swelling of the nodes is obvious clinically. They are tender or painful, often show inflammation of the overlying skin, when an actual abscess exists, typically perforate and discharge pus.

Oral Manifestation

Tuberculous lesions of oral cavity are relatively uncommon. Oral lesions are seldom primary, but rather are secondary to pulmonary disease. It appears most likely that the organisms are carried in the sputum and enter the mucosal tissue through a small break in the surface. It is possible that the organisms may be carried to the oral tissues by a hematogenous route to be deposited in the

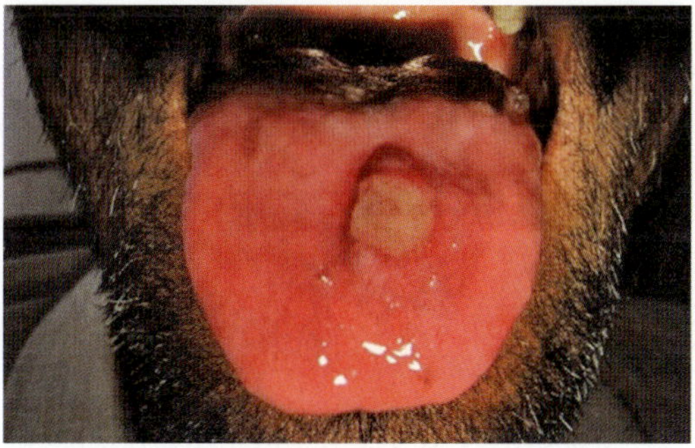

Fig. 12.1

submucosa and subsequently to proliferate and ulcerate the overlying mucosa. Tongue is most commonly affected, followed by the palate, lips, buccal mucosa, gingiva and frenula. Ulcer is irregular, superficial or deep, painful ulcer which tends to increase slowly in size. Tuberculosis may also involve the maxilla or mandible, periapical inflammation by way of bloodstream produce tuberculous periapical granuloma or tuberculoma.

Diagnosis

Diagnosis of active infection must be confirmed by demonstration of the organisms by special microbial stains and culture of infected tissue or sputum. The presence of acid fast bacilli (AFB) in sputum smear is the gold standard for diagnosis for TB.

Tuberculin Test

The mantoux test involves subcutaneous injection of 0.1 ml of 5 tuberculin units of purified protein derivative of siebert stabilized with tween 80 or 1 tuberculin unit of PPDRT 23 into the forearm. It is positive if indurations is seen after 48–72 hours. The maximum diameter of the induration measured by palpation and not redness, and interpreted as follows:

More than 15 mm or ulceration	–	Strongly positive
More than 10 mm	–	Positive
5–9 mm	–	Indeterminate
Less than 5 mm	–	Nsegative

The tuberculin skin test has greater value in excluding tuberculosis than in diagnosing it.

Treatment

Multiple drug therapy is often recommended as *M.tuberculosis* mutates and resists single drug therapy, Isoniazid (INH) combined with rifampicin for nine months or INH, rifampicin and pyrazinamide for two months followed by INH and rifampicin for four months. Other drugs used are streptomycin and ethambutol.

FUNGAL DISEASES

Candidiasis

Candidiasis is caused by a yeast-like fungus, candida albicans. Old age is one of the predisposing factor for candidiasis.

Chronic Atrophic Candidiasis (Denture Stromatitis)

It is a candida associated lesion. It is also known as denture sore mouth, a diffuse erythema and edema of denture-bearing area, often occurring with angular cheilitis. Usually asymptomatic except for the soreness and the presenting complaint may be angular stomatitis. Mandibular mucosa is rarely affected. Denture related candidiasis may be the most common form of the oral disease.

Treatment

Suspensions of nystatin, held in contact with the oral lesions. The other drugs of value are clotrimazole amphotericin B and miconazole.

Phycomycosis (Mucormycosis, Zygomycosis)

Phycomycosis is a fungal infection caused by the order mucorales. It is also especially common in patients with diabetic mellitus, especially those with diabetic ketoacidosis.

Clinical Features

Two main types of phycomycosis infection occur in human being— (1) superficial and (2) visceral, although sometimes it is also classified as localized and disseminated. The superficial infection includes involvement of the external ear, the fingernails and the skin. The visceral forms of phycomycosis are of three main types: (a) Pulmonary, (b) gastrointestinal, (c) rhinocerebral.

Infections of the head by these organisms are characterized by the classical syndrome of uncontrolled diabetes, cellulitis, ophthalmoplegia and meningoencephalitis.

One early clinical manifestation of the disease is the appearance of a reddish-black nasal turbinate and septum with a nasal discharge. The necrosis may extend to the paranasal sinuses and orbital cavity, with the development of sinus tracts and slouging of tissue. Cases of phycomycosis involving the maxillary sinus may present clinically as a mass in the maxilla, resembling carcinoma of the antrum and X-rays may support the latter diagnosis.

Treatment and Prognosis

Control of predisposing factors such as diabetes surgical excision, if the lesion is localized and administration of amphotericin B, since it is the only drug with proven efficacy.

DIABETES MELLITUS

Diabetes mellitus is a metabolic disease characterized by dysregulation of carbohydrate, protein and lipid metabolism. The primary feature of this disorder is elevation in blood glucose levels (hyperglycemia), resulting from either a defect in insulin secretion from the pancreas, a change in insulin action or both.

Sustained hyperglycemia has been shown to affect almost all tissues in the body and is associated with significant complications of multiple organ systems including the eyes, nerves, kidneys, and blood vessels. These complications are responsible for the high degree of morbidity and mortality seen in the diabetic population.

Classification

The most common forms of diabetes are termed type I and type II (Table 12.1). Type I was previously called insulin-dependent

Table 12.1: Classification of diabetes mellitus

Type I	(Insulin-dependent diabetes, juvenile diabetes)
Type II	(Non-insulin dependent diabetes, adult-onset diabetes)
Gestational diabetes (pregnancy diabetes)	
Other types of diabetes • Genetic defects affecting Beta-cell function or insulin action • Pancreatic diseases or injuries (pancreatic cancer, pancreatitis, traumatic injury, cystic fibrosis, pancreatectomy) • Infections (congenital rubella, cytomegalovirus infection) • Drug induced diabetes (steroid hormones, thyroid hormones) • Endocrine disorder (hyperthyroidism, Cushing's syndrome, acromegaly, pheochromocytoma) • Other genetic syndrome (with associated diabetes)	

diabetes mellitus or juvenile diabetes while type II diabetes was formerly known as non-insulin dependent diabetes or adult onset diabetes.

Both insulin-dependent and non-insulin dependent diabetes individuals may take insulin as part of their management regimen. The difference is that type I patients are truly dependent on insulin therapy, whereas type II patients may benefit from insulin therapy but are not dependent on it for survival.

Gestational diabetes occurs during pregnancy and usually resolves after delivery. Other types may occur in individuals with certain genetic disorders, pancreatic diseases, infections, injuries to the pancreas and endocrine diseases. Drug therapy with certain agents may also induce a diabetic state.

Clinical Presentations and Diagnosis

The onset of type I diabetes is usually abrupt, whereas type II diabetes is often present for years without overt signs or symptoms. Patients with undiagnosed diabetes may present with one or more signs and symptoms. The diagnosis of diabetes is based on the presence of clinical signs and symptoms along with specific laboratory findings.

Both fasting and non-fasting plasma glucose test provide a determination of glucose levels at a single moment in time, namely at the time the blood sample is collected.

Complications

The major cause of the high morbidity and mortality rate associated with diabetes is a group of microvascular and macrovascular complications affecting multiple organ systems.

People with diabetes have a greatly increased risk for blindness, kidney failure, myocardial infarction, stroke, and necessary limb amputation. The onset and progression of these complications are strongly linked to the presence of sustained hyperglycemia. The complication rate and severity of complications increases. Other disorders such as hypertension and dyslipidemia commonly seen in people with diabetes increase the risk for microvascular and macrovascular complications. There may also be genetic determinants of risk for diabetic complications (Table 12.2).

Table 12.2: Complications of diabetes

• Retinopathy	•	Vision changes Blindness	
• Nephropathy	•	Renal failure	
• Neuropathy	•	Sensory	– Loss of sensation in hands and feet – Impotence – Other sensory dysfunction
	•	Autonomic	– Gastroparesis
	•	Changes in cardiac rate, rhythm, conduction	– Other autonomic dysfunction
	•	Macrovascular diseases	– Peripheral vascular disease – Coronary artery disease – Cardiovascular (stroke)
	•	Alterations in wound healing	

Management

Primary treatment goals for diabetes patients include the achieving of blood glucose levels that are close to normal as possible and the prevention of diabetic complications.

Diet, exercise, weight control and medications are the mainstays of diabetic care.

Oral agents—sulfonylureas, metformin, thiazolidinedione agents.

Insulin

All type I diabetic patients use exogenous insulin, as do many with type II diabetes. Insulin is taken via subcutaneous injection most often with a syringe.

Oral Consideration

Oral conditions that are seen in individuals with diabetes may include burning mouth, altered wound healing, and an increased incidence of infection. Enlargement of parotid glands and xerostomia can occur.

Medications that diabetic patients often take for related or unrelated systemic conditions may have significant xerostomic effects. Neuropathy of the autonomic system can also cause changes in salivary secretion since salivary flow is controlled by the sympathetic and parasympathetic pathways. Dry mucosal surfaces are easily irritated and are associated with 'burning mouth' syndrome and also provide a favorable environment for the growth of fungal organisms.

Periodontal Health and Diabetes

Diabetes is a risk factor for the prevalence and severity of gingivitis and periodontitis. Diabetes is associated with increased gingival inflammation in response to bacterial plaque, but the degree of glycemic control is an important variable in this relationship. Diabetes not only increases the prevalence and severity of periodontitis but also the progression of bone loss and attachment loss over time.

Periodontitis is similar to the classic complications of diabetes in its variation among individuals. Progressive destructive periodontitis is also more common in those with poor control.

Hyperglycemia results in increased gingival crevicular fluid glucose levels, which may significantly alter periodontal wound-healing events by changing the interaction between cells and their extra cellular matrix within the periodontium. Vascular changes seen in retina, glomerulus and perineural areas also occur in the periodontium.

Diabetes results in changes in the function of host defense cells such as polymorphonuclear neutrophils adherence, chemotaxis and phagocytosis are impaired. Defects in this first line of defense against periodontopathic microorganisms may significantly increase periodontal destruction.

Dental Management of the Diabetic Patients

Glycemic control appears to play an important role in the response to periodontal therapy. Well-controlled diabetic patients with periodontitis have positive responses to non-surgical therapy, periodontal surgery and maintenance that are similar to those of people without diabetes.

In undiagnosed diabetic patients findings such as enlarged gingival tissue that bleed easily upon manipulation and the presence of multiple periodontal abscess. The determination of patient's recent glycosylated hemoglobin values provides a measure of glycemic control over the preceding 2 to 3 months. HbA_{1C}values of less than 8% indicate relatively good glycemic control and values greater than 10% indicate poor control. The dental treatment considerations for diabetic patients include stress reduction, treatment setting the use of antibiotics, diet modification, appointment timings, changes in medication regimen and management of emergencies.

Elevation of epinephrine and cortisol happen during stressful situation and these hormones elevate blood glucose levels. The small amounts of epinephrine in dental local anesthetics at 1/1,00,000 concentration have no significant effect on blood glucose. Conscious sedation should be considered for extremely anxious patients.

Prophylactic antibiotic coverage prior to surgical therapy if the diabetic patient's glycemic control is poor. This usually applies to emergency situation since elective procedures are generally deferred until glycemic control improves. Diet is major component of diabetes management, diet alterations that are made because of dental treatment may have a major impact on the patient. Another diet change occurs when patients are placed on orders to take nothing by mouth (NPO) before dental treatment, a common recommendation before conscious sedation.

It is generally best to plan dental treatment to either before or after periods of peak insulin activity. For those who take insulin, the greatest risk of hypoglycemia will occur about 30 to 90 minutes after injecting Lisproinsulin, 2 to 3 hours after regular insulin and 4 to 10 hours after NPH or Lente insulin. For those who taking oral sulfonylureas, peak insulin activity depends on the individual drug taken. Metformin and thiazolidinediones rarely cause hypoclycemia. Clinician must be aware that the patient is at risk for perioperative hypoglycemia. It is helpful to check the pretreatment blood glucose level and to have a source of carbohydrates readily available.

Emergencies in Diabetic Patients

Most common diabetic emergency is hypoglycemia, a potentially life-threatening complication. Signs and symptoms include confusion, sweating, tremors, agitation, anxiety, dizziness, tingling or numbness and tachycardia. Severe hypoglycemia may result in seizures or loss of consciousness. The patient should be given 15 gm of oral carbohydrate in form that will be rapidly absorbed following check of blood glucose level. Intravenous line of 25 to 50 ml of 50% dextrose given if patient is unable to take by oral route.

In some instances hyperglycemia may mimick hypoglycemia. If glucometer is not available, these can be treated as hypoglycemia because small amount of extra glucose desired from treatment will not have significant effect, whereas if glucose-elevating emergency is thought and treatment is withheld from a patient, severe adverse outcomes are possible. Hyperglycemia develops more slowly than does hypoglycemia. Diabetic ketoacidosis and hyperosmolar non-ketotic acidosis require immediate medical evaluation and treatment.

The intimate relationship between oral health and systemic health and systemic health in diabetics needs interaction between dental and medical professionals. Oral health assessment and treatment should become as common as the eye, foot and kidney evaluations that are routinely performed as part of preventive medical therapies.

13

Endocrine Diseases

THYROID HORMONE

Hypothyroidism

A failure of thyrotrophic function on the part of the pituitary gland or an atrophy or destruction of the thyroid gland per se leads to an inability of the thyroid to produce sufficient hormone to meet the requirements of the body. In adults it is referred to as myxedema and it is not a rare disease.

Clinical Features

The clinical and orofacial finding in myxedematous patients are apparently limited to the soft tissues of the face and mouth. The lips, nose, eyelids and suborbital tissues are edematous and swollen. The tongue is large and edematous, frequently interfering with speech.

The myxedematous swelling is probably an extravascular, extracellular accumulation of water and protein in the tissues. The protein has a greater osmotic effect than the serum proteins, accounting for the increased blood protein concentration and decreased plasma volume which are found in myxedema.

Diagnosis

It is usually based on history, clinical and laboratory assessment and hormonal assays.

Hyperthyroidism

Hyperthyroidism has been described into two fundamentally different types.

- *Exophthalmic goiter:* Characterized by diffuse hyperplasia of the thyroid and by eye signs.

- *Toxic adenoma:* Hyperfunctions originates in a benign tumor of the thyroid gland.

Most of the symptoms of hyperthyroidism are due to an increased metabolic activity of the tissues of the body. This is usually manifested as an increased basal metabolic rate. The serum protein-bound iodine concentration is elevated. The urinary iodine excretion is reduced because of the increased iodine uptake by the thyroid gland.

Clinical Features

Patient may exhibit tremor, tachycardia, sweating, weight loss, nervousness, muscle weakness, heat intolerance and exophthalmic goiter. Patients suffering from hyperthyroidism usually present a facial expression of surprise or excitement with wide-eyed staring such patients are nervous and highly emotional, they have increased sensitivity to epinephrine and are usually hypertensive.

Diagnosis

Thyroid function tests are useful to determine hyperthyroidism. Other tests include radioactive iodine uptake, free thyroid assay, free thyroxine index and total serum thyroxine estimation.

PARATHYROID HORMONE

Parathyroid glands release parathormone that maintains plasma ionized calcium level. Two well-defined clinical entities are associated with parathyroid glands—hyperparathyroidism, which manifests its symptoms primarily in the bones and the kidneys and hypoparathyroid tetany.

Secondary Hyperparathyroidism

Hyperparathyroidism can also occur secondary to other disorders, the most common being end-stage renal diseases. It is reported in chronic renal failure patients.

Clinical Features

Pathologic fracture may be the first symptom of the disease, although bone pain and joint stiffness are early symptoms. The loss of phosphorous and calcium in this disturbance results in a generalized osteoporosis with abortive attempts at bone repair and new bone formation. The new bone may be resorbed and the resorption may lead to pseudocyst formation, the extent of which depends on the duration and intensity of the disease.

Radiographically, bones of affected persons show a general radiolucency as compared with those of normal people. Later sharply defined round or oral radiolucent areas develop, which may be lobulated.

If such lobulated lesion develops in the mandible, it must be carefully differentiated from ameloblastoma which frequently has the same appearance. In the jaws, the radiograph in hyperparathyroidism has been described as having a 'ground glass' appearance. The lamina dura around the teeth may be partially lost.

Diagnosis

It is confirmed by blood investigation which shows hypercalcemia, hypophosphatemia and elevated serum parathormone level along with hypercalciuria and hyperphosphaturia. The serum alkaline phosphates level is increased in osteolytic lesions.

Treatment

Excision of parathyroid tumor will cure the patient. Multiple tumors may develop over an extended period of time, patients who have had one parathyroid tumor should be followed for life.

PITUITARY GROUP OF HORMONES

The pituitary is considered the master gland of the body.

Hypopituitarism

Hypopituitarism is caused by compression or atrophy of anterior pituitary cells or defect in the hypothalamic control of hormonal secretion.

Clinical Features

The typical evidences of hypopituitarism resulting in pituitary dwarfism are a diminutive but well-proportional body, fine, silky, sparse hair on the head and other hairy region, wrinkled atrophic skin and often hypogonadism.

Hypopituitarism in the adult is usually due to an infraction of the pituitary called Simmond's diseases. It is characterized by loss of weight and diminished sexual function. The basal metabolic rate is markedly lowered and since Simmond's disease represents a panhypopituitarism, there is a decrease in the activity of the many hormones of the pituitary gland and of those glands that are under pituitary regulation. Changes in the head include thin eyebrows, loss of eyelashes, sharp features, thin lips and an immobile expression. There will be an immobile expression. There will be a decreased salivary flow due to hypo functioning of salivary gland which leads to increased caries activity and periodontal disease.

Hyperpituitarism

An increase in the number of granules in the acidophilic cells or an adenoma of the anterior lobe of the pituitary is associated with gigantism or acromegaly. If the increase occurs before the epiphyses of the long bones are closed, gigantism results, if the increase occurs later in life, i.e. after epiphyseal closure, acromegaly develops.

Clinical Features

Gigantism is characterized by a general symmetric overgrowth of the body, some persons with this disturbance attaining a height of over 8 feet. Later in life such people usually show genital underdevelopment and excessive perspiration and they complain of headache, lassitude, fatigue, muscle and joint pains and hot flashed. It is also characterized by the presence of broad, enlarged nose, thick and furrowed oily skin. Organomegaly and hypertension are common findings. Skeletal changes include frontal bossing and prognathic mandible. Increased glove, ring and shoe size indicates the changes in the hands and feet. Hypercementosis is a common finding in the intraoral radiographs.

Diagnosis

Radiographic features suggestive of hyperpituitarism include enlarges sella turcica, enlarges paranasal sinuses, tufted terminal phalanges and widened carpal joint spaces. Also, patients will have abnormal glucose tolerance hypertension and hyperphosphatemia.

Adrenal Hormones

Adrenal glands are small, paired endocrine glands, situated at the posterosuperior poles of the kidneys. They have an outer cortex and inner medulla, which secrete various hormones,

- Adrenal cortex is divided into
- *Zona glomerulosa:* Secretes mineralocorticoids (e.g. aldosterone)
- *Zona fasciculate:* Secretes glucocorticoids and cortisol
- *Zona reticularis:* Secretes sex hormones

Chronic Insufficiency of the Adrenal Cortex: Addison's diseases

It develops usually following the autoimmune destruction of adrenal glands and frequently occurs in conjunction with other autoimmune disorders.

Clinical Features

Early manifestations include lethargy, fatigue and muscular weakness that may persist for months. Patient feels tired after minimal exertion but feels well on walking. Feeble heart action, general debility, vomiting, diarrhea and severe anemia are also seen.

Hypoglycemia, dehydration, hypertension, elevated serum potassium and postural dizziness develop following low blood levels of cortisol.

Hyperfunction of Adrenal Gland

Adrenogenital syndrome: A condition known as adrenogenital syndrome results when hyperplasia or tumors of the adrenal cortex occur. Depending on the age of onset and the gender of the person affected, the clinical signs are pseudohermaphroditism, sexual precocity and hirtuism in women or feminization in men.

Cushing's syndrome: This syndrome is a result of hormonal excess resulting from any of the following

- Hyperplastic adrenal cortices without any other clinically evident endocrine lesion.
- Adrenal cortical adenoma or carcinoma.

- Ectopically located adrenal-like tumor, e.g. of an ovary
- ACTH : Secreting tumor of the anterior pituitary associated with adrenal cortical hyperplasia.
- Nonpituitary carcinoma, e.g. of a lung or the pancreas, with secretion of an ACTH: like material that induces adrenal cortical hyperplasia.

When the syndrome is associated with spontaneous bilateral adrenal hyperplasia, it is referred to as Cushing's disease. It is characterized by a rapidly acquired adiposity about the upper portion of the body, mooning of the face, a tendency to become round-shouldered and develop a buffalo hump at the base of neck, alteration in hair distribution, muscle weakness, vascular hypertension, glycosuria not controlled by insulin and albuminuria.

14

Neuromuscular Diseases

Diseases that affect both nerve and muscle tissue encompass a broad range of symptoms that often have profound implications for successful management of the dental patient.

CEREBROVASCULAR DISEASE

Cerebrovascular disease includes all disorders that cause damage to blood vessels supplying the brain, thereby producing neurologic damage, stroke and cerebrovascular accident (CVA) are terms used to describe an acute neurologic injury resulting from a severe interruption in the flow of blood to the brain. Complete cessation of flow may render an irreversible cerebral infarct within a period of 3 to 4 minutes. General symptoms following stroke include variable motor paralysis, sensory loss, visual difficulties, and speech impairment.

CEREBROVASCULAR ACCIDENT OR STROKE

Approximately 80% of strokes are associated with the development of atherosclerosis leading to cerebral ischemia and infarction. The remaining 20% of cases are caused by cerebral hemorrhage.

CEREBRAL INFARCTION

A cerebral infarction occurs when there is ischemia and necrosis of an area of the brain after a reduction of blood supply to a level below the level necessary for cell survival. The two major causes of cerebral infarction are thrombosis and embolism, often the result of atherosclerosis.

The resulting deficit depends on the particular vessel involved and the extent of any collateral circulation. Thromboembolic cerebral infarction also occurs as a complication of other diseases. Many of the emboli that occlude intracranial vessels arise from thrombi that have formed in the left side of the heart. Emboli originating from the heart are often the result of thrombus formation after acute myocardial infarction, chronic atrial fibrillation or rheumatic heart disease. Hypertension is an important risk factor in the development of thrombosis, particularly at the carotid bifurcation.

CEREBRAL HEMORRHAGE

Hemorrhage of intracranial vessels may also cause stroke. The two most common reasons for hemorrhage are (1) rupture of an aneurysm and (2) an arteriovenous malformation that hemorrhage spontaneously, often secondary to hypertension or following the administration of anticoagulant medication.

The majority of cases are aneurysmal. Aneurysms are localized dilations of arteries, caused by structural weakness of vessel walls.

Clinical Manifestations of Stroke

Strokes due to ischemia may be classified clinically either as a stroke in evolution or as a completed stroke. 'Stroke in evolution' is a descriptive term used to indicate a condition in which symptoms associated with cerebral ischemia become progressively worse while the patient is under observation.

A complete stroke caused by a thrombus often evolves slowly and the full neurologic picture may take hours or even days to emerge. This clinical picture commonly includes hemiplegia, aphasia, and cranial nerve defects involving nerves V, VII, IX, and X.

Oral Considerations

The first line of medical management of stroke patients is often anti-coagulant therapy; the patient may have a predisposition to excessive bleeding. In addition, it may be necessary to confer with the patient's physician to obtain current coagulation values so as to ensure that the patient is stable for more invasive dental treatment.

Xerostomia is a common side effect of the medication used in the management of cerebrovascular disease and related disease processes. Patients who are thus affected can then be susceptible to a higher caries rate.

Meticulous oral hygiene, more frequent recalls, saliva substitutes, and fluoride application can aid in maintenance of the dentition.

Stroke patients can also have physical disabilities, which can affect the orofacial area and can alter the provision of dental care. Patients with weakness in the muscles of the orofacial region may have poor control of oral secretions, a reduced gag reflex and changes in their ability to masticate, leading to poor nutrition. Patients with apraxia affecting the orofacial region may have impaired voluntary movements, such as protruding the tongue, expectorating, and lip puckering.

Careful history taking, checking of blood pressure prior to treatment, avoidance of lengthy appointments, and general reassurance are all important factors in the provision of dental treatment for patients with a history of stroke.

MULTIPLE SCLEROSIS

Multiple sclerosis is a chronic neurologic disease associated with the demyelination of axons within the central nervous system. The disease occurs more frequently among women. The disease presents in the form of recurrent attacks, in some cases, the attacks are years apart. The most common symptoms following an acute exacerbation include impairment of vision, muscular incoordination and bladder dysfunction.

Clinical Manifestations

The clinical signs and symptoms of multiple sclerosis depend on the site of demyelinating lesion. The lesions may occur almost anywhere in the central nervous system, but they have a predilection for certain areas. More than 60% of individuals have visual disturbances caused by demyelinated lesions of the second cranial nerve. The loss of vision usually occurs over a period of several days, with partial recovery within 1 month. Other ophthalmic symptoms include 'color blindness' and diplopia caused by involvement of third, fourth and sixth cranial nerves.

Weakness or paresthesia of the extremities, with an increase in the deep tendon reflexes, is another common early finding in cases of multiple sclerosis.

An important feature of motor nerve function in multiple sclerosis is the relative fluctuation of symptoms on a daily basis. These symptoms may remit for long periods and then suddenly reverse, leading to paraplegia. Other common signs of the disease include bladder dysfunction, euphoria, ataxia, vertigo and generalized incoordination.

Oral Considerations

Certain clinical manifestation of multiple sclerosis affect the orofacial region, three are of particular interest to the dentist, trigeminal neuralgia, sensory neuropathy of the trigeminal nerve and facial palsy.

Trigeminal neuralgia is present in about 2% of cases of multiple sclerosis. Pain is normally severe and lancinating, but trigger zones may be absent. In time, the pain often becomes less severe but more continuous. Effective drug therapy includes the use of carbamazepine, baclofen, gabapentin or phenytoin. When medication proves inadequate, thermocoagulation, surgical sectioning of the nerve or alcohol injection may be considered.

Sensory neuropathy secondary to multiple sclerosis can be progressive and difficult to diagnosis. It most often affects the second and third divisions of the trigeminal nerve, has a sudden onset, and is painful. Neuropathy to the mental nerve can cause numbness of the lower lip and chin.

Facial paralysis appears later in the course of the disease. It may be difficult to distinguish between the paralysis caused by multiple sclerosis and that due to Bell's palsy, but up to 24% of multiple sclerosis sufferers may experience facial paralysis.

PARKINSONISM (PARKINSON'S DISEASES, PARALYSIS AGITANS)

Parkinsonism is a neurodegenerative disorder characterized by rigidity, tremors, bradykinesia and impaired postural reflexes.

The most common form of parkinsonism is Parkinson's disease (paralysis agitans), but parkinsonism is seen in variety of disorders such as postencephalitic parkinsonism, arteriosclerotic parkinsonism and post-traumatic parkinsonism following close head injury affects adults in the middle or late life. The rate of prevalence is higher in those who are older than 60 years of age.

Clinical Manifestations

Tremor, rigidity, bradykinesia and postural instability are the cardinal features of parkinsonism and may be present in any combination. The tremor is most conspicuous at rest, is enhanced by emotional stress, and tends to be less severe during voluntary activity. Rigidity (increase in resistance to passive movement) is responsible for the characteristically flexed posture seen in many patients. The most disabling symptoms are due to bradykinesia, manifested as a slowness of voluntary movement and a reduction in automatic movements such as the swinging of the arms while walking.

The onset of the disease is generally insidious. Mild stiffness of the muscles of the extremities and tremor of the hands are frequently early signs. The typical hand tremor is often called a "pill-rolling" movement, characterized by the rubbing of the thumb against the fingers and is particularly pronounced when the patient is otherwise at rest. The general stiffness progresses slowly until significant disability is noted by the patient. Walking becomes more difficult and patient develops a slow shuffling gait with a stooped position. As the ability to perform voluntary movements decreases, patient usually experience an inability to coordinate separate or independent movements.

Many of the signs of Parkinson's disease are found in the head and neck. The typical 'mask like' facial appearance with infrequent blinking and lack of expression is caused by bradykinesia. The muscle rigidity also causes difficulty in swallowing, resulting in drooling. Speech becomes labored because of the lack of muscle control and mandibular tremor results in masticatory results, especially in those with removable dental appliances. Abnormalities in oral behavior, such as purposeless chewing, grinding and sucking movements are also well recognized in patients with Parkinson's disease and make dental treatment especially difficult.

Oral Considerations

Patients must be treated in upright position, making access to certain areas of the oral cavity difficulty for the dentist. In addition, anxiety in a Parkinson's disease patient can increase both the tremor and degree of muscle rigidity.

Due to dysphagia and an altered gag reflex, special precautions must be taken to avoid the aspiration of water or materials used during dental procedures. In patients who suffer with hypersialorrhea, maintaining a dry field in procedures that require such can be especially difficult. Xerostomia on the other hand is a common side effect on antiparkinsonism medications the consequent root caries and recurrent decay must be treated. Patients also often have difficulty in maintaining their dentition because of their physical disability. When dental treatment is finished the patient should be warned to take care when moving from a supine position since levodopa has a significant orthostatic hypotensive effect.

EPILEPSY

Epilepsy is a condition characterized by abnormal, recurrent, and excessive neuronal discharges precipitated by many different disturbances within the central nervous system. These aberrant discharges may cause episodes of sensory and motor abnormalities as well as loss of consciousness. Each episode of aberrant neurologic activity is referred to as a seizure.

Epilepsy in older adults is more often associated with cerebrovascular diseases such as stroke and tumor.

Clinical Manifestations

Nonspecific changes such as headache, mood alterations, lethargy and myoclonic jerking alert some patients to an impending seizure hours before it occurs. These prodromal symptoms are distinct from the aura that may precede a generalized seizure by a few seconds or minutes and that is itself a part of the attack, arising locally from a restricted region of the brain.

The most common type of seizure is the tonic-clonic or grand mal seizure; 90% of epileptics experience it alone or in combination with another type of seizure. A grand mal seizure characteristically begins with an aura. The aura may be experienced as epigastric discomfort, as an emotion, or as a hallucination of hearing, vision, or smell. The aura is followed seconds to minutes later by consciousness, a cry, and tonic muscle spasms, this rigid phase lasts about 30 seconds. Because of spasm of respiratory muscles, the patient does not breathe and become cyanotic during this period. The tonic phase is followed by a clonic phase composed of convulsive jerky movements, incontinence, and tongue biting. The patient may injure him or herself seriously if he or she is near hard or sharp objects.

Oral Considerations

Medical history should indicate what type of seizure the patient has, how well the seizures are controlled, the frequency, and duration of seizures, the potential triggers for seizures and what to expect if the patient has a seizure.

As a general rule, it is better to place a fixed prosthesis rather than a removable appliance because of the potential for removable appliances to become dislodged during a seizure.

Patients under anticonvulsant drugs are subject to gingival enlargement. Most often associated with patients taking phenytoin. Clinically phenytoin gingival overgrowth starts in the interdental papillae and occurs only where teeth are present. The papillae enlarge bucally and lingually. The best treatment of phenytoin gingival overgrowth begins with prevention soon after being placed on anticonvulsant therapy, each patient should be referred to a dentist for oral hygiene instruction and gingival curettage. Gingivectomy can be done for patients who have not been properly managed and who develop gross gingival enlargement.

Other side effects on taking phenytoin include megaloblastic anemia, hirsutism and lymphadenopathy.

15 Oral Tumors

EPITHELIAL TUMORS

Benign Epithelial Tumors

Verruciform Xanthoma

Verruciform xanthoma is a hyperplastic condition of the epithelium of the mouth, skin, and genitalia, with a characteristic accumulation of lipid laden histiocytes beneath the epithelium. First reported in 1971, it remains largely an oral disease; its cause is still unknown. Although verruciform xanthoma is a papillary lesion, human papilloma virus does not appear to play a role in its pathogenesis. The lesion probably represents an unusual reaction or immune response to localized epithelial trauma or damage.

Clinical Features

Verruciform xanthoma is typically seen in whites, 40 to 70 years of age. There is a strong female predilection (1:2 male-to-female ratio). Approximately half of the intraoral lesions occur on the gingiva and alveolar mucosa, but any oral site may be involved. The lesion appears as a well-demarcated, soft, painless, sessile, slightly elevated mass with a white, yellow-white, or red color and a papillary or roughened (verruciform) surface. Rarely, flat - topped nodules are seen without surface projections. Most lesions are smaller than 2 cm in greatest diameter; no oral lesion larger than 4 cm has been reported. Multiple lesions occasionally have been described. Clinically, verruciform xanthoma may be similar to squamous papilloma, condyloma acuminatum, or early carcinoma.

Treatment and Prognosis

The verruciform xanthoma is treated with conservative surgical excision. Recurrence after removal of the lesion is rare, and no malignant transformation has been reported.

Epulis Fissuratum (Inflammatory Fibrous Hyperplasia; Denture Injury Tumor and Denture Epulis)

The epulis fissuratum is a tumor like hyperplasia of fibrous connective tissue that develops in association with the flange of an ill fitting complete or partial denture.

Clinical Features

The epulis fissuratum typically appears as a single or multiple fold or folds of hyperplastic tissue in the alveolar vestibule. Most often, there are two folds of tissue, and the flange of the associated denture fits conveniently into the fissure between the folds. The redundant tissue is usually firm and fibrous, although some lesions appear erythematous and ulcerated. The size of the lesion can vary from localized hyperplasias less than 1 cm in size to massive lesions that involve most of the length of the vestibule. The epulis fissuratum usually develops on the facial aspect of the alveolar ridge, although occasional lesions are seen lingual to the mandibular alveolar ridge. The epulis fissuratum most often occurs in middle aged and older adults, as would be expected with a denture-related lesion. It may occur on either the maxilla or mandible. The anterior portion of the jaws is affected much more often than the posterior areas. There is a pronounced female predilection; another similar but less common fibrous hyperplasia, often called a fibroepithelial polyp or leaf like denture fibroma, occurs on the hard palate beneath a maxillary denture. This characteristic lesion is a flattened pink mass that is attached to the palate by a narrow stalk. Usually, the flattened mass is closely applied to the palate and sits in a slightly cupped out depression. However, it is easily lifted up with a probe, which demonstrates its pedunculated nature. The edge of the lesion often is serrated and resembles a leaf.

Treatment and Prognosis

The treatment of the epulis fissuratum or fibroepithelial polyp consists of surgical removal, with microscopic examination of the excised tissue. The ill fitting denture should be remade or relined to prevent a recurrence of the lesion.

Papillary Hyperplasia (Denture Papillomatosis)

Inflammatory papillary hyperplasia is a reactive tissue growth that usually, although not always, develops beneath a denture. The condition most often appears to be related to the following:

- An ill-fitting denture
- Poor denture hygiene
- Wearing the denture 24 hours a day

Candida also has been suggested as a cause, but any possible role appears uncertain.

Clinical Features

Inflammatory papillary hyperplasia usually occurs on the hard palate beneath a denture base. Early lesions may involve only the palatal vault, although advanced cases cover most of the palate. Less frequently, this hyperplasia develops on the edentulous mandibular alveolar ridge or on the surface of an epulis fissuratum. On rare occasions, the condition occurs on the palate of a patient without a denture, especially in people who habitually breathe through their mouth or have a high palatal vault.

Candida-associated palatal papillary hyperplasia also has been reported in dentate patients with human immunodeficiency virus (HIV) infection. Inflammatory papillary hyperplasia is usually asymptomatic. The mucosa is erythematous and has a pebbly or papillary surface. Many cases are associated with denture stomatitis.

The mucosa in inflammatory papillary hyperplasia exhibits numerous papillary growths on the surface that are covered by hyperplastic stratified squamous epithelium. In advanced cases, this hyperplasia is pseudoepitheliomatous in appearance.

The connective tissue can vary from loose and edematous to densely collagenized. A chronic inflammatory cell infiltrate is usually seen, which consists of lymphocytes and plasma cells. Less frequently, polymorphonuclear leukocytes are also present. If underlying salivary glands are present, they often show sclerosing sialadenitis.

Treatment and Prognosis

For very early lesions of inflammatory papillary hyperplasia, removal of the denture may allow the erythema and oedema to subside, and the tissues may resume a more normal appearance. The condition also may show improvement after topical or systemic antifungal therapy. For more advanced and collagenized lesions, many clinicians prefer to excise the hyperplastic tissue before fabricating a new denture. Various surgical methods have been used, including the following:

- Partial thickness or full-thickness surgical blade excision
- Curettage
- Electro surgery
- Cryosurgery

After healing, the patient should be encouraged to leave the new denture out at night and to keep it clean.

Sebaceous Hyperplasia

Sebaceous hyperplasia is characterized by a localized proliferation of sebaceous glands of the skin.

Clinical Features

Cutaneous sebaceous hyperplasia usually affects adults older than 40 years of age. It occurs most commonly on the skin of the face, especially the cheeks and forehead, and is characterized by one or more soft non tender papules with white, yellow or normal coloration. Lesions are usually umbilicated with a small central depression. Representing the area where the ducts of the involved sebaceous lobules terminate. Most lesions arc smaller than 5 mm in greatest diameter and take considerable time to reach even this small size. Compression of the lesion usually causes sebum. The thick yellow-white product of the sebaceous gland, to be expressed in the central depressed area. This feature helps clinically to distinguish sebaceous hyperplasia from basal cell carcinoma. An oral counterpart, which probably has no relation to the skin lesion, appears as a white to yellow papule or nodular mass with a "cauliflower" appearance, usually of the buccal mucosa.

Treatment and Prognosis

No treatment is necessary for sebaceous hyperplasia except for aesthetic reason. Excisional biopsy is curative.

Actinic Lentigo (Lentigo Solaris; Solar Lentigo; Age Spot; Liver Spot and Senile Lentigo)

Actinic lentigo is a benign brown macule that results from chronic ultraviolet light damage to the skin. It is found in more than 90% of whites older than 70 years of age and rarely is seen before age 40. It does not occur within the mouth but is seen frequently on the facial skin.

Clinical Features

Actinic lentigo is common on the dorsa of the hands, on the face, and on the arms of elderly whites. It is typically multiple, but individual lesions appear as uniformly pigmented brown to tan macules with well-demarcated but irregular borders. Although the lesion may reach more than 1 cm in diameter, most examples are smaller than 5 mm. Adjacent lesions may coalesce, and new ones continuously arise with age. Unlike ephelides, no change in color intensity is seen after exposure to ultraviolet light.

Treatment and Prognosis

No treatment is required for actinic lentigo, except for aesthetic reasons.

Oral Melanotic Macule (Focal Melanosis)

The oral melanotic macule is a flat, brown mucosal discoloration produced by a focal increase in melanin deposition and possibly a concomitant increase in the number of melanocytes. The cause remains unclear. Unlike the cutaneous ephelis (freckle), the melanotic macule is not dependent on sun exposure.

Clinical Features

The oral melanotic macule occurs at any age in both men and women; however, biopsy samples demonstrate a 2:1 female predilection. The vermilion zone of the lower lip is the most common site of occurrence (33%), followed by the buccal mucosa, gingiva, and palate. The typical lesion appears as a solitary (17% are multiple), well-demarcated, uniformly tan to dark-brown, asymptomatic, round or oval macule with a diameter of 7 mm or smaller. Occasional lesions may be blue or black. Lesions are not reported to enlarge after diagnosis, which suggests that the maximum dimension is achieved rather rapidly and remains constant thereafter.

Treatment and Prognosis

Treatment is usually not required for the melanotic macule, except for aesthetic considerations.

Premalignant Lesions

Leukoplakia (Leukokeratosis)

Oral leukoplakia *(leuko* = white; *plakia* = patch) is defined by the World Health Organization (WHO) as "a white patch or plaque that cannot be characterized clinically or pathologically as any other disease." The term is strictly a clinical one and does not imply a specific histopathologic tissue alteration. Although leukoplakia is not associated with a specific histopathologic diagnosis, it is typically considered to be a precancerous or premalignant lesion. When the outcome of a large number of leukoplakic lesions is reviewed, the frequency of transformation into malignancy is greater than the risk associated with normal or unaltered mucosa.

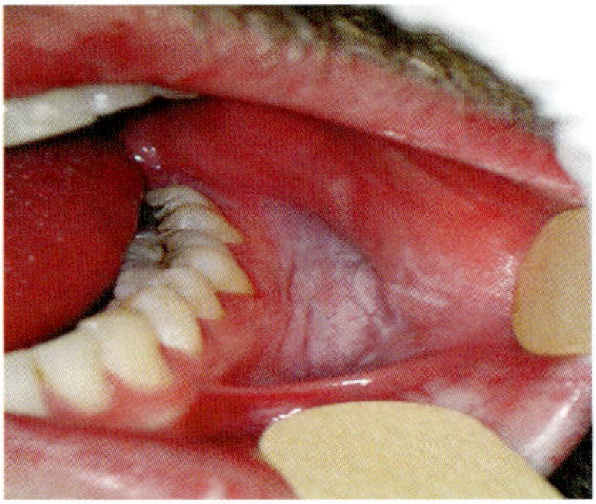

Fig. 15.1: Leukoplakia

Incidence and Prevalence

Although leukoplakia is considered a premalignant lesion, the use of the clinical term in no way suggests that histopathologic features of epithelial dysplasia are present in all lesions. Dysplastic epithelium or frankly invasive carcinoma is, in fact, found in only 5 to 25% of biopsy samples of leukoplakia. Leukoplakia is by far the most common oral pre cancer, representing 85% of such lesions.

Etiology

The cause of leukoplakia remains unknown, although hypothesis tells tobacco, alcohol, sanguinaria, ultraviolet radiation, microorganisms such as treponema pallidum, candida albicans, human papilloma virus and trauma are most commonly associated with leukoplakia development.

Clinical Features

Leukoplakia usually affects persons older than 40 years of age. Prevalence increases rapidly with age, especially for males, and as many as 8% of men older than 70 years of age reportedly are affected Approximately 70% of oral leukoplakias are found on the lip vermilion, buccal mucosa, and gingival lesions on the tongue, lip vermilion, and oral floor, however, account for more than 90% of those that show dysplasia or carcinoma. Mild or thin leukoplakia, which seldom shows dysplasia on biopsy, may disappear or continue unchanged, for tobacco smokers who do not reduce their habit, as many as two thirds of such lesions slowly extend laterally, become thicker, and acquire a distinctly white appearance. The affected mucosa may be leathery to palpation, and fissures may deepen and become more numerous. At this stage or phase, the lesion is often called a homogeneous or thick leukoplakia. Most thick, smooth lesions remain indefinitely at this stage. Some, perhaps as many as one third, regress or disappear; a few become even more severe, develop increased surface irregularities, and are then called granular or nodular leukoplakia, Some lesions demonstrate sharp or blunt projections and have been called verrucous or verruciform leukoplakia. Leukoplakia may become dysplastic, even invasive, with no change in its clinical appearance. However, some lesions eventually demonstrate scattered patches of redness, called erythroplakia. Such areas usually represent sites in which epithelial cells are so immature or atrophic that they can no longer produce keratin. This intermixed red-and-white lesion, called erythroleukoplakia or speckled leukoplakia, represents a pattern of leukoplakia that frequently reveals advanced dysplasia upon biopsy.

Treatment and Prognosis

Because leukoplakia represents a clinical term only, the first step in treatment is to arrive at a definitive histopathologic diagnosis. Therefore, a biopsy is mandatory and will guide the course of treatment. Some smoking- related leukoplakias with no or minimal dysplasia may disappear or diminishing size within 3 months after the patient stops smoking. Thus, habit cessation is recommended. Chemo prevention also may be useful, but remains primarily experimental.

Erythroplakia (Erythroplasia; Erythroplasia of Queyrat)

As with leukoplakia, erythroplakia is defined as a red patch that cannot be clinically or pathologically diagnosed as any other condition. Erythroplakia also may occur in conjunction with leukoplakia and has been found concurrently with a large proportion of early invasive oral carcinomas. Although erythroplakia is less common than leukoplakia, it has a much greater potential to be severely dysplastic at the time of biopsy or to develop invasive malignancy at a later time.

Clinical Features

Erythroplakia is predominantly a disease of older men, with a peak prevalence at 65 to 74 years. The floor of mouth, tongue, and soft palate are the most common sites of involvement, and multiple lesions may be present. The altered mucosa appears as a well-demarcated erythematous macule or plaque with a soft, velvety texture. It is usually asymptomatic and may be associated with an adjacent leukoplakia (erythroleukoplakia). Nonspecific mucositis, candidiasis, psoriasis or vascular lesions may clinically mimic erythroplakia, and biopsy often is required to distinguish between them.

Treatment and Prognosis

Red lesions of the oral mucosa, especially those of the oral floor and ventral or lateral tongue, should be viewed with suspicion, and a biopsy should be performed. If a source of irritation can be identified and removed, biopsy of such a lesion may be delayed for 2 weeks to allow a clinically similar inflammatory lesion time to regress.

Nicotine Stomatitis (Nicotinepalatinus; Smoker's Palate)

Once a common mucosal change of the hard palate, nicotine stomatitis has become less common as cigar and pipe smoking have lost popularity. Although this lesion is a white keratotic change obviously associated with tobacco smoking. It does not appear to have a premalignant nature, perhaps because it develops in response to heat rather than the chemicals in tobacco smoke. Because pipe smoking generates more heat on the palate than other forms of smoking, nicotine stomatitis has been associated most often with this habit. Similar changes can also be produced by the longterm use of extremely hot beverages.

Clinical Features

Nicotine stomatitis most commonly is found in men older than 45 years of age. With long-term exposure to heat, the palatal mucosa becomes diffusely gray or white, numerous slightly elevated papules are noted, usually with punctuate red centres. Such papules represent inflamed minor salivary glands and their ductal orifices. The mucosa that covers the papules frequently appears whiter than the surrounding epithelium. The palatal keratin may become so thickened that a fissured or "dried mud" appearance is imparted. The whiteness usually involves marginal gingiva and interdental papillae and leukoplakia of the buccal mucosa is occasionally seen. A heavy brown or black tobacco stain may be present on the teeth.

Treatment and Prognosis

Nicotine stomatitis is completely reversible. Even when it has been present for many decades. The palate returns to normal, usually within 1 to 2 weeks of smoking cessation.

Malignant Epithelial Tumors

Squamous Cell Carcinoma

It is the sixth most common cancer in males and the twelfth most common in females. In some countries, such as India, it is the most common cancer. Approximately 94% of all oral malignancies are squamous cell carcinoma. The overall male-to-female gender ratio is 3:1.

Etiology of Oral Cancer

The cause of oral squamous cell carcinoma is multifactorial. No single causative agent or factor (carcinogen) has been clearly defined or accepted, but both extrinsic and intrinsic factors may be at work. It is likely that more than a single factor is needed to produce such a malignancy (cocarcinogenesis). Extrinsic factors include such external agents as tobacco smoke, smokeless tobacco, betel quid, alcohol, phenolic agents, radiation, syphilis, and (for vermilion cancers only) sunlight. Intrinsic factors include systemic or generalized states, such as general malnutrition or iron-deficiency anemia. Heredity does not appear to play a major causative role in oral carcinoma. Many oral squamous cell carcinomas have been documented to be associated with or preceded by a precancerous lesion,

Clinical and Radiographic Features

Persons with oral squamous cell carcinoma are most often older men who have been aware of an alteration in an oral cancer site for 4 to 8 months before seeking professional help (8 to 24 months among lower socioeconomicgroups). There is minimal pain during the early growth phase, and this may explain the delay in seeking professional care. If the health care professional does not have a high index of suspicion. An additional several weeks or months may elapse before a biopsy is performed. Oral squamous cell carcinoma has a varied clinical presentation including:

- Exophytic (mass-forming; fungating, papillary, verruciform)
- Endophytic (Invasive, burrowing, ulcerated)
- Leukoplakic (white patch)
- Erythroplakic (red patch)
- Erythroleukoplakic (Combined red-and-whit e patch)

The leukoplakic and erythroplakic: examples are probably early cases that have not yet produced a mass or ulceration and the clinical features are identical to those described for premalignant leukoplakia and erythroplakia. These mucosal surface changes typically are destroyed by the developing exophytic or endophytic carcinoma, but many cases are diagnosed before their complete destruction and show residual precancerous lesions involving adjacent mucosa. An exophytic lesion typically has a surface that is irregular, fungating, papillary, or verruciform and its color may vary from normal to red to white. Depending on the amount of keratin and vascularity. The surface is often ulcerated, and the tumor feels hard (indurated) on palpation. The endophytic growth pattern is characterized by a depressed, irregularly shaped, ulcerated, central area with a surrounding "rolled" border of normal red or white mucosa. The rolled border results from invasion of the tumor downward and laterally under adjacent epithelium. disease. Destruction of underlying bone when present, may be painful or completely painless, and it appears on radiographs as a " moth-eaten" radiolucency with ill defined or ragged margins (an appearance similar to osteomyelitis). Carcinoma also can extend for many centimeters along a nerve (perineural invasion) without breaking away to form a true metastasis.

Metastasis

The metastatic spread of oral squamous cell carcinoma is largely through the lymphatics to the ipsilateral cervical lymph nodes. A cervical lymph node that contains a metastatic deposit of carcinoma is usually firm to stony hard, nontender, and enlarged. If the malignant cells have perforated the capsule of the node and invaded into surrounding tissues. The node will feel "fixed " or not easily movable. Occasionally, contra lateral or bilateral metastatic deposits are seen, and at least 2% of patients have distant (below the clavicles) metastasis at diagnosis; in some studies this figure is as high as 22%. The most common sites of distant metastasis are the lungs, liver and bones, but any part of the body may be affected. Carcinoma of the lower lip and oral floor tends to travel to the submental nodes; tumors from the posterior portions of the mouth travel to the superior jugular and digastric nodes. Lymphatic drainage from the oropharynx leads to the jugulodigastric chain of lymph nodes or to the retropharyngeal nodes, and metastatic deposits from oropharyngeal carcinoma are usually found there.

Treatment and Prognosis

Carcinoma of the vermilion zone of the lip is usually treated by surgical excision typically a wedge resection, with excellent results. Only 8% recur and 5-year survival rates are 95 to 100%. In one study that evaluated all vermilion cancers diagnosed in a population over 6 decades, not one patient died of his or her disease. Squamous cell carcinomas of the upper lip vermilion appear to have a different biologic behavior than do those of the lower lip. The treatment of intraoral squamous cell carcinoma is guided by the clinical stage of the disease and consists of wide (radical) surgical excision. Radiation therapy or a combination of surgery and radiation therapy, tumor's location may influence the treatment plan. Oropharyngeal lesions usually receive radiation therapy. A variety of chemotherapeutic agents are used as adjunctive therapy; some can temporarily reduce the size of a tumor mass, but none has improved survival rates significantly.

Verrucous Carcinoma (Snuff Dipper's Cancer; Ackerman's Tumor)

Verrucous carcinoma is a low-grade variant of oral squamous cell carcinoma. Reported first by Ackerman in 1948 as a spit tobacco-associated malignancy. It has been diagnosed since then at several extraoral sites, including laryngeal, vaginal and rectal mucosa and skin from the breast axilla, ear canal and soles of the feet. Tumors at anatomic sites other than the mouth are unrelated to tobacco use. Several investigators have identified HPV subtypes 16 and 18 in some oral verrucous carcinomas, but the significance of this is unclear. Many verrucous carcinomas arise from the oral mucosa in people who chronically use chewing tobacco or snuff. Typically in the area where the tobacco is habitually placed.

Clinical Features

Verrucous carcinoma is found predominantly in men older than 55 years of age (average age, 65 to 70 years), in areas where women are frequent users of spit tobacco; However, elderly females may predominate. The most common sites of oral mucosal involvement include the mandibular vestibule, the buccal mucosa and the hard palate. The site of occurrence often corresponds to the site of chronic tobacco placement. In cultural groups who keep spit tobacco in the maxillary vestibule or under the tongue, these locations are the most commonly involved sites. Oral verrucous carcinoma is usually extensive by the time of diagnosis, and it is not unusual for a tumor to be present in the mouth for 2 to 3 years before definitive diagnosis.

The lesion appears as a diffuse, well demarcated, painless, thick plaque with papillary or verruciform surface projections. Lesions are typically white but also may appear erythematous or pink. The color depends on the amount of keratin produced and the degree of host inflammatory response to the tumor. Leukoplakia or tobacco pouch keratosis may be seen on adjacent mucosal surfaces and verrucous carcinoma is a lesion that may develop from the high-risk precancer, proliferative verrucous leukoplakia (PVL). Both PVL and verrucous carcinoma may have been reported in the past by the name oral florid papillomatosis.

Treatment and Prognosis

Because metastasis is an extremely rare event in verrucous carcinoma, the treatment of choice is surgical excision without radical neck dissection.

Spindle Cell Carcinoma (Sarcomatoid Squamous Cell Carcinoma; Polypoid Squamous Cell Carcinoma)

Spindle cell carcinoma is a rare variant of squamous cell carcinoma characterized by dysplastic surface squamous epithelium in conjunction with an invasive spindle cell element. It may be indistinguishable from connective tissue sarcomas or other spindle cell malignancies at the level of the light microscope. In the past, this biphasic lesion was thought to be a "collision" tumor between a carcinoma and sarcoma, but most authorities now consider the spindle cells to be simply an anaplastic type of carcinoma cell.

Clinical Features

The mean age at diagnosis for spindle cell carcinoma is 57 years (range: 29 to 93 years), There is no sex predilection, the neoplasm occurs predominantly in the upper aerodigestive tract, especially the larynx, oral cavity, and esophagus, Within the mouth, the lower lip, lateral posterior tongue, and alveolar ridges are common sites, but other areas may be involved. In contrast to other oral cancers, the spindle cell carcinoma typically appears as a pedunculated, polypoid mass, but it may occasionally appear as a sessile, nodular or fungating mass, or an ulcer. Pain and paresthesia are prominent features.

Treatment and Prognosis

The treatment of choice for spindle cell carcinoma is radical surgery, with neck dissection when clinically positive nodes are present. Radiotherapy and chemotherapy are ineffective.

Adenosquamous Carcinoma

Adenosquamous carcinoma is a rare variant of squamous cell carcinoma that is characterized histopathologically by a combination of adenocarcinoma and squamous cell carcinoma. The adenoid (glandular) pattern, which includes mucus production, has been demonstrated clearly in metastatic deposits. Some authorities consider this carcinoma to be merely a high-grade mucoepidermoid carcinoma.

Clinical Features

Cases of adenosquamous carcinoma have been reported from the tongue, oral floor, and other mucosal surfaces, usually in older adults, There is no sex predilection, The clinical appearance is that of a painless, nodular, broad-based mass with or without surface ulceration, Eighty percent of patients have metastatic deposits with in the neck nodes at diagnosis.

Treatment and Prognosis

Radical surgical excision, with or without radiation therapy, is the treatment of choice for patients with adenosquamous carcinoma. The prognosis is poor, with 60% of patients dying of disease, usually within 2 years of diagnosis.

Basaloid Squamous Carcinoma (Basaloid Squamous Cell Carcinoma)

Basaloid squamous carcinoma is a lesion found primarily in the upper aerodigestive tract mucosa and represents the most recently described variant of squamous cell carcinoma, It has a tendency to develop in the hypopharynx, but dozens of oral lesions have been reported.

Clinical Features

Basaloid squamous carcinoma occurs predominantly in men, in persons 40 to 85 years of age, and in abusers of alcohol and smoked tobacco. It occurs most commonly in the larynx and tongue base, but any region of the upper aerodigestive tract may be affected, The individual lesion clinically appears as a fungating mass or ulcer and maybe painful or interfere with swallowing (dysphagia), almost 80% of patients have cervical metastasis at the time of diagnosis of this high-grade, aggressive cancer.

Treatment and Prognosis

Basaloid squamous carcinoma is an aggressive malignancy, affected patients have a mean survival time of only 23 months. Surgery followed by radiotherapy is the recommended treatment. Usually with adjuvant chemotherapy for the distant metastases.

Carcinoma of the Maxillary Sinus

Carcinoma of the maxillary sinus or antrum is an uncommon malignancy of unknown cause. It does not appear to be related to sinusitis, nasal polyps, or tobacco use. Most lesions remain asymptomatic for long periods while the tumor grows to fill the sinus. Therefore, the diagnosis may not be made until the lesion has perforated through the surrounding bone.

Clinical and Radiographic Features

Typically, carcinoma of the maxillary sinus is a disease of elderly persons. There is a slight predilection for males. More than 80% of cases are advanced (stage III and stage IV) at the time of diagnosis, affected patients generally complain of a chronic unilateral nasal stuffiness or notice an ulceration or mass of the hard palate or alveolar bone. When the second division of the trigeminal nerve is involved, intense pain or paresthesia of the mid face or maxilla may occur, perhaps simulating a toothache, Teeth in the area of the tumor may become loosened, and dental radiographs often reveal a "moth eaten" destruction of the lamina dura and surrounding bone. A panoramic radiograph shows a cloudy sinus with destruction of its bony wall, although the extent of the tumor is visualized best by computed tomography (CT) or magnetic resonance imaging (MRI).

If the tumor perforates the lateral wall of the sinus, unilateral facial swelling and pain are usually present. If the extension is medial, nasal obstruction or hemorrhage usually occurs. Extension superiorly results in displacement or protrusion of the eyeball. Approximately 4% of patients have cervical or submandibular lymph node metastasis at the time of diagnosis. Distant metastasis is quite uncommon until late in the progression of disease.

Treatment and Prognosis

Carcinoma confined within the maxillary sinus is treated by hemi maxillectomy; those that have perforated through the surrounding bone are treated by radiotherapy or combined radical surgery and radiotherapy.

Nasopharyngeal Carcinoma

Nasopharyngeal carcinoma refers to a group of malignancies that arise from the lining epithelium of the lymphoid tissue-rich nasopharynx; similar tumors are found in the palatine tonsil and base of tongue. These three anatomic sites are collectively called waldeyer's tonsillar tissue or waldeyer's ring. Nasopharyngeal carcinoma is rare in most areas of the world. Infection with Epstein-Barr virus, environment, diets deficient in vitamin C, and consumption of salt fish that contains potentially carcinogenic N-nitrosamines have been implicated as contributory factors.

Clinical Features

Nasopharyngeal carcinoma occurs in all age groups. It also occurs three times more commonly in men than in women. The primary lesion, which usually arises from the lateral nasopharyngeal wall, often is small and difficult to detect, even when the area is examined endoscopically. The first sign of disease for 50 to 60% of patient is an enlarged, firm to hard, cervical lymph node, which represents metastatic tumor. Symptoms related to the ear are described by slightly less than half of these patients. If the tumor arises near the eustachian tube, unilateral serous otitis media, otalgia, or hearing loss from obstruction may be the presenting complaint. Epistaxis, nasal obstruction, and pharyngeal pain may be present. The tumor may invade through the foramen lacerum in to the brain, producing central nervous system (CNS) symptoms, or it may involve cranial nerves in the area, causing specific symptoms related to those nerves. Significantly, 5 to 10% of patients also have distant metastasis at the time of diagnosis.

Treatment and Prognosis

Because of the inaccessibility of the nasopharynx and the high frequency of metastasis at diagnosis, nasopharyngeal carcinoma is treated most frequently with radio therapy to the nasopharynx and neck. This may be combined with chemotherapy, but this addition has not been shown to improve survival. The prognosis ranges from good to poor. depending on the stage of the disease.

Basal Cell Carcinoma (Basal Cell Epithelioma; Rodent Ulcer)

Basal cell carcinoma, the most common skin cancer (and the most common of all cancers), is a locally invasive, slowly spreading primary epithelial malignancy that arises from the basal cell layer of the skin and its appendages This cancer results from chronic exposure to ultraviolet radiation.

Clinical Features

Basal cell carcinoma is a disease of adult whites, especially those with fair complexions. Although most patients are older than 40 years of age at the time of diagnosis. The most common form of this lesion, the nodular (noduloulcerative) basal cell carcinoma. Begins as a firm. painless papule that slowly enlarges and gradually develops a central depression and an umbilicated appearance. One or more telangiectatic blood vessels are usually seen coursing over the rolled border surrounding the central depression. When the lesion is pressed, a characteristic pearly opalescent quality is discerned. Expanding ulceration often develops in the central depressed area and the patient may give a history of intermittent bleeding followed by healing. Untreated lesions continue to enlarge slowly over months and years, with ulceration and destruction of underlying structures, hence their historical name, rodent ulcer. Destruction of underlying bone or cartilage may occur, but metastasis is extremely rare. Several other clinicopathologic varieties of this tumor have also been described. Pigmented basal cell carcinoma is seen occasionally and represents a noduloulcerative tumor colonized by benign melanocytes. The melanin production imparts a tan, brown, black, or even bluish color to the lesion, and usually the pigment is not distributed uniformly as it would be in amelanocytic nevus.

Sclerosing (morpheaform basal cell carcinoma) is an insidious lesion that often mimics scar tissue. The overlying skin appears pale and atrophic and the lesion is firm to palpation with poorly demarcated borders. A slight elevation may be noted at the edges of the tumor. Often a great deal of invasion has occurred before the patient becomes aware of a problem. The superficial basal cell carcinoma occurs primarily on the skin of the trunk. Often, lesions are multiple and appear as well-demarcated, erythematous. Scaly patches that may be mistaken clinically for psoriasis. A fine, elevated, "thread like" border is seen at the margins. Some investigators believe that the basal cell carcinoma associated with the nevoid basal cell carcinoma syndrome should be placed in a separate category. These lesions develop in both sun-exposed and protected areas of the skin and may number in the hundreds on a single patient. The tumors associated with this syndrome usually do not produce a significant degree of tissue destruction.

Treatment and Prognosis

The treatment of basal cell carcinoma often depends on the size and site of the lesion. Small lesions 1cm are treated by routine surgical excision, laser ablation, or electrodesiccation and curettage, with 5 mm margins of clinically normal appearing skin beyond the visible lesion. These methods result in a cure rate of 95 to 98%. Radical surgical excision and radiation therapy are recommended for large or aggressive lesions. For sclerosing type lesions, recurrent lesions or lesions situated near embryonic planes of fusion (along which these tumor cells lend to invade), a procedure called Mohsmicrographic surgery should be used.

Merkel Cell Carcinoma (Merkel Cell Tumor; Neuroendocrine Carcinoma of Skin; Small Cell Carcinoma of skin and Trabecular Carcinoma of Skin)

The Merkel cell carcinoma first described in 1972, is a rare, aggressive primary malignancy with neuroendocrine features. It occurs primarily on the skin of the head and neck region. Lesional cells contain cytoplasmic granules that resemble the neurosecretory granules found within the epidermal Merkel cells of touch receptor regions. Intraoral and lip vermilion cases have been reported but are rare.

Clinical Features

Merkel cell carcinoma typically appears in older people. It occurs primarily on the sun exposed areas of fair skinned individuals. Most commonly all the skin of the face. The vermilion border of the lower lip is also a susceptible site. The tumor usually appears as a slowly enlarging dome-shaped nodule with a smooth surface and prominent surface vessels (telangiectasias), It is red or violaceous and ranges in size from 0.5 to 5.0 cm. Ulceration rarely is seen. Occasional lesions grow rapidly, and 25% demonstrate local metastasis at diagnosis, being its innocuous clinical appearance.

Treatment and Prognosis

Merkel cell carcinoma is treated with wide local excision, which is combined with lymph node dissection when clinically palpable nodes are found. The addition of postoperative radiotherapy improves the prognosis.

Melanoma (Malignant Melanoma; Melanocarcinoma)

Melanoma is a malignant neoplasm of melanocytic origin that arises from a benign melanocytic lesion or de novo from melanocytes within otherwise normal skin or mucosa. Although most melanomas occur on the skin, they may develop at any site where melanocytes are present. Damage from ultraviolet radiation is considered a major causative factor, as suggested by the fact that the incidence of melanoma increases for light-complexioned populations as they approach the equator, but chronic sun exposure does not seem to be as significant as *it* is for other cutaneous cancers, such as basal and squamous cell carcinoma. Acute sun damage may be of greater causative importance than chronic exposure in melanoma. Lesions of the intraoral mucosa, of course, are not related to sun exposure. The risk of melanoma development is two to eight times greater when a relative has a history of the cancer. The mucosal melanoma tends to appear at a higher stage and is much more aggressive than its cutaneous counterpart. At least one in three patients with oral melanoma have a history of a pigmented macule in the region of the tumor for some time before melanoma diagnosis. Melanoma occasionally affects the parotid gland, usually as a metastatic deposit from a scalp, conjunctival or paranasal tumor.

Clinical Features

Most melanomas are seen in white adults. The average age of affected persons is 50 to 55 years. But cases are rather evenly distributed over the 30 to 80 year age group. Four clinicopathologic types of melanoma have been described:

1. Superficial spreading melanoma
2. Nodular melanoma
3. Lentigo maligna melanoma
4. Acral lentiginous melanoma

Melanomas tend to exhibit two directional patterns of growth: (1) The radial growth phase and (2) the vertical growth phase. In the early stages of melanoma development, the radial growth phase lends to predominate in lentigo maligna melanoma, superficial spreading melanoma, and acral lentiginous melanoma. In these lesions, the malignant melanocytes tend to spread horizontally through the basal layer of the epidermis. Eventually, however, the malignant cells begin to invade the underlying connective tissue, thus initiating the vertical growth phase. With nodular melanoma, the radial growth phase is very short or nonexistent and the vertical growth phase predominates. Because many clinical similarities exist between melanoma and its benign counterpart, the melanocytic nevus, an "ABCD" system of evaluation has been developed to help distinguish a melanoma clinically from a melanocytic nevus.

The "ABCD" clinical features of melanoma

- Asymmetry (because of its uncontrolled growth pattern)
- Border irregularity (often with notching)
- Color variegation (which varies from shades of brown to black, white, red, and blue, depending on the amount and depth of melanin pigmentation)
- Diameter greater than 6 mm (diameter)

Superficial spreading melanoma: Superficial spreading melanoma is the most common form of melanoma, representing 70% of cutaneous lesions. The most common sites of origin are the interscapular area of males and the back of the legs of females. This form of melanoma appears as a macule with a variety of potential colors (i.e. tan, brown, gray, black, blue, white, pink). Typically, the lesion is smaller than 3 cm in greatest diameter at diagnosis, but it may be several times that size. Many lesions are slightly elevated. Clinically, invasion is indicated by the appearance of surface nodules or induration, and usually occurs within 1 year of discovery of the precursor macule. Satellite macules or nodules of malignant cells may develop around the primary lesion.

Nodular melanoma: Nodular melanoma represents 15% of cutaneous melanomas, and one third of such lesions develop in the head and neck area. Nodular melanoma is thought to begin almost immediately in the vertical growth phase and, therefore, typically appears as a nodular elevation that rapidly invades into the connective tissue. Nodular melanoma is usually a deeply pigmented exophytic lesion, although sometimes the melanoma cells are so poorly differentiated that they no longer can produce melanin, resulting in a non-pigmented amelanotic melanoma.

Lentigo maligna melanoma: Lentigo maligna melanoma, which accounts for 5 to 10% of cutaneous melnomas, develops from a precursor lesion called lentigo maligna (Hutchinson's freckle). Lentigo maligna occurs almost exclusively on the sun-exposed skin of fair complexioned elderly persons, particularly in the midfacial region, and represents a melanoma *in situ* in a purely radial growth phase. The lesion appears as a large, slowly expanding macule with irregular borders and a variety of colors, including tan, brown, black, and even white. Patients usually indicate that the lesion has been present and has slowly expanded laterally for years. The average duration of the radial growth phase is 15 years. The appearance of nodularity within a lentigomaligna signals the onset of the invasive or vertical growth phase and the transition to lentigomaligna melanoma.

It typically develops on the palms of the hands, soles of the feet, subungual area and mucous membranes. It begins as a darkly pigmented, irregularly marginated macule, which later develops a nodular invasive growth phase. Recently, some authorities have separated this lesion into two entities:

1. Acral lentiginous melanoma and
2. Mucosal lentiginous melanoma.

Oral melanoma is often nodular at the time of diagnosis, but early lesions may be flat. Affected persons are usually in their sixth or seventh decade of life. Two-thirds of patients are male. Four of every five oral melanomas are found on the hard palate or maxillary alveolus. An oral lesion typically begins as a brown to black macule with irregular borders. The macule extends laterally and a lobulated exophytic mass develops once the vertical growth is initiated. Ulceration may develop early, but many lesions are dark, lobulated, exophytic masses without ulceration at the time of diagnosis. More than 20% of oral melanomas contain so little pigment that they have an essentially normal mucosal tint. Pain is nota common feature except in ulcerated lesions, and most lesions remain relatively soft to palpation. Underlying or adjacent bone may show radiographic evidence of irregular or "moth-eaten" destruction.

Treatment and Prognosis

Microscopic measurement of the depth of invasion is an important component of the histopathologic evaluation of melanoma because of its correlation with the prognosis. Surgical excision is the only curative treatment, although the extent of the excision is somewhat controversial. Older literature suggests that surgical margins of 3 to 5 cm around the tumor are necessary to achieve control, regardless of the site of the lesion. More recent studies indicate that a 1cm margin is adequate for small, early tumors. For larger, more deeply invasive tumors, wide surgical excision still is recommended. Surgical removal of regional lymph nodes is recommended for lesions with a histopathologic depth of invasion that exceeds 1.24 mm. Radiation therapy has no significant impact on survival. Although adjunct chemotherapy and immunotherapy are showing promise.

Connective Tissue Tumors

Malignant Fibrous Histiocytoma

The malignant fibrous histiocytoma is a sarcoma with both fibroblastic and histiocytic features. Although this term was first introduced in 1963. This tumor is now considered to be the most common soft tissue sarcoma in adults.

Clinical Features

The malignant fibrous histiocytoma is primarily a tumor of older age groups. The most common complaint is an expanding mass that may or may not be painful or ulcerated. Tumors of the nasal cavity and paranasal sinuses produce obstructive symptoms.

Treatment and Prognosis

The malignant fibrous histiocytoma is an aggressive tumor that is usually treated by radical surgical resection.

Fibrous Histiocytoma

Fibrous histiocytomas are a diverse group of tumors that exhibit both fibroblastic and histiocytic differentiation. Although the cell of origin is still uncertain, it may arise from the tissue histiocyte, which then assumes fibroblastic properties.

Clinical Features

The fibrous histiocytoma can develop almost anywhere in the body. The most common site is the skin of the extremities, where the lesion is called a dermatofibroma. Tumors of the oral and perioral region are uncommon. Although oral tumors can occur at any site. The most frequent location is the buccal mucosa and vestibule. Rare intrabony lesions of the jaws have also been reported. Oral fibrous histiocytomas tend to occur in middle-aged and older adults. The tumor is usually a painless nodular mass and can vary in size from a few millimeters to *several* centimeters in diameter.

Treatment and Prognosis

Local surgical excision is the treatment of choice. Recurrence is uncommon on, especially for superficial tumors. Larger lesions of the deeper soft tissues have a greater potential to recur.

Lipoma

The lipoma is a benign tumor of fat. Although it represents by far the most common mesenchymal neoplasm. Most examples occur on the trunk and proximal portions of the extremities. Lipomas of the oral and maxillofacial region are much less frequent. The pathogenesis of lipomas is uncertain, but they appear to be more common in obese people. However, the metabolism of lipomas is completely independent of the normal body fat. If the caloric intake is reduced, lipomas do not decrease in size, although normal body fat may be lost.

Clinical Features

Oral lipomas are usually soft, smooth-surfaced nodular masses that can be sessile or pedunculated. Typically, the tumor is asymptomatic and often has been noted for many months or years before diagnosis. Most are less than 3 cm in size, but occasional lesions can become much larger. Although a subtle or more obvious yellow hue often is detected clinically, deeper examples may appear pink. The buccal mucosa and buccal vestibule are the most common intraoral sites and account for 50% of all cases. Some buccal cases may not represent true tumors, but rather herniation of the buccal fat pad, which may occur subsequent to surgical removal of third molars. Less common sites include the tongue, floor of the mouth, and lips. Most patients are 40 years of age or older. Although lipomas elsewhere in the body are reported to be twice as common in females as in males. Oral lipomas are characterized by a more balanced sex distribution.

The angiolipoma consists of an admixture of mature fat and numerous small blood vessels.

Myxoid lipomas exhibit a mucoid background and may be confused with myxoid liposarcomas.

The spindle cell lipoma demonstrates variable amounts of uniform appearing spindle cells in conjunction with a more typical lipomatous component.

Pleomorphic lipomas are characterized by the presence of spindle cells plus bizarre, hyperchromatic giant cells; they can be difficult to distinguish from apleomorphic liposarcoma.

Intramuscular (infiltrating) lipomas often are more deeply situated and have an infiltrative growth pattern that extends between skeletal muscle bundles.

Treatment and Prognosis

Lipomas are treated by conservative local excision, and recurrence is rare.

Tumors of Nerve Tissue

Traumatic Neuroma (Amputation Neuroma)

The traumatic neuroma is not a true neoplasm but a reactive proliferation of neural tissue after transection or other damage of a nerve bundle. After a nerve has been damaged or severed, the proximal portion attempts to regenerate and reestablish innervation of the distal segment by the growth of axons through tubes of proliferating Schwann cells. If these regenerating elements encounter scar tissue or otherwise cannot reestablish innervation. A tumor like mass may develop at the site of injury.

Clinical and Radiographic Features

Traumatic neuromas of the oral mucosa are typically smooth-surfaced, non ulcerated nodules. They can develop at any location but are most common in the mental foramen area, tongue and lower lip. A history of trauma often can be elicited; some lesions arise subsequent to tooth extraction or other surgical procedures. Intraosseous traumatic neuromas may demonstrate a radiolucent defect on oral radiographs. Traumatic neuromas can occur at any age, but they are diagnosed most often in middle aged adults. They appear to be slightly more common in females. Although pain has been traditionally considered a hallmark of this lesion, studies indicate that only one fourth to one third of oral traumatic neuromas are painful. This pain can be intermittent or constant and ranges from mild tenderness or burning to severe radiating pain. Neuromas of the mental nerve are frequently painful, especially when impinged on by a denture or palpated.

Treatment and Prognosis

The treatment of choice for the patient with a traumatic neuroma is surgical excision, including a small portion of the involved nerve bundle. Most lesions do not recur; in some cases, however the pain persists or returns at a later date

Palisaded Encapsulated Neuroma (solitary Circumscribed Neuroma)

The palisaded encapsulated neuroma is a benign neural tumor with distinctive clinical and histopathologic features. Although it was first recognized only as recently as 1972, it represents one of the more common superficial nerve tumors, especially in the head and neck region. The cause is uncertain, but some authors have speculated that trauma may play an etiologic role; the tumor is generally considered to represent a reactive lesion rather than a true neoplasm.

Clinical Features

The palisaded encapsulated neuroma shows a striking predilection for the face. The nose and cheek are the most common specific sites. The lesion is most frequently diagnosed between the fifth and seventh decades of life, although the tumor often has been present for many months or years. It is a smooth-surfaced, painless dome shaped papule or nodule that is usually less than 1 cm in diameter. There is no sex predilection. Oral palisaded encapsulated neuromas are not uncommon, although many are probably diagnosed microscopically as neurofibromas or neurilemomas. The lesion appears most frequently on the hard palate and maxillary labial mucosa, although it also may occur in other oral locations.

Treatment and Prognosis

The treatment for the palisaded encapsulated neuroma consists of conservative local surgical excision. Recurrence is rare.

Neurilemoma (Schwannoma)

The neurilemmoma is a benign neural neoplasm of Schwann cell origin.

Clinical and Radiographic Features

The neurilemoma is a slow-growing, encapsulated tumor that typically arises in association with a nerve trunk. As it grows, it pushes the nerve aside. Usually, the mass is asymptomatic, although tenderness or pain may occur in some instances. The lesion is most common middle-aged adults and can range from a few millimeters to several centimeters in size. The tongue is the most common location for oral neurilemmomas. Although the tumor can occur almost anywhere in the mouth. On occasion, the tumor arises centrally within bone and may produce bony expansion. Intraosseous examples are most common in the posterior mandible and usually appear as either unilocular or multilocular radiolucencies on radiographs. Pain and paresthesia are not unusual for intrabony tumors.

Tumors of Vascular Origin

Hemangiopericytoma

The hemangiopericytoma is a rare neoplasm that is presumably derived from pericytes, (i.e. cells whose processes encircle the endothelial cells of capillaries).

Clinical Features

Hemangiopericytomas are seen primarily in adults. Tumor is usually a slow-growing, painless mass. Superficial lesions may demonstrate vascular pigmentation. A distinctive form of hemangiopericytoma (hemangiopericytoma-like tumor) occurs in the nasal cavity and paranasal sinuses. The lesion primarily occurs in middle aged and older adults and usually results in symptoms of nasal obstruction or epistaxis.

The hemangiopericytoma is usually fairly well circumscribed and exhibits tightly packed cells that surround endothelium-lined vascular channels. The cells are haphazardly arranged and demonstrate round to ovoid nuclei and indistinct cytoplasmic borders, occasionally they are spindle-shaped. The blood vessels often show irregular branching, which results in a characteristic "stag horn" and "antler like" appearance.

Treatment and Prognosis

For hemangiopericytomas with a benign histopathologic appearance local excision is the treatment of choice, more extensive surgery is required for tumors with malignant characteristics.

Tumors of Muscle Origin

Leiomyoma

Leiomyomas are benign tumors of smooth muscle that most commonly occur in the uterus, gastrointestinal tract, and skin. Leiomyomas of the oral cavity are rare. Most of these probably have their origin from vascular smooth muscle.

The three types are:

1. Solid leiomyomas
2. Vascular leiomyomas (angiomyomas or angioleiomyomas)
3. Epithelioid leiomyomas (leiomyoblastomas)

Clinical and Radiographic Features

The oral leiomyoma can occur at any age and is usually a slow-growing firm mucosal nodule. Most lesions are asymptomatic, although occasional tumors can be painful. Solid leiomyomas are typically normal in color, although angiomyomas may exhibit a bluish hue. The most common sites are the lips, tongue, palate, and cheek, which together account for 80% of cases. Extremely rare intraosseous examples may present as unilocular radiolucencies of the jaws.

Treatment and Prognosis

Oral leiomyomas are treated by local surgical excision. The lesion should not recur.

Rhabdomyoma

Benign neoplasms of skeletal muscle are called rhabdomyomas. Rhabdomyomas of the head and neck can be subclassified into two major categories. Adult and fetal rhabdomyomas.

Clinical Features

Adult rhabdomyomas of the head and neck occur primarily in middle-aged and older patients, with about 70% of cases found in men. The most frequent sites are the pharynx, oral cavity and larynx. Intraoral lesions are most common in the floor of the mouth, Soft palate and base of tongue. The tumor appears as a nodule or mass that can grow to many centimeters before discovery and Laryngeal and pharyngeal lesions often lead to airway obstruction. Sometimes, the tumor is multinodular in nature, with two or more discrete nodules found in the same anatomic location. Occasional cases are multicentric, with separate distinct tumors at different sites.

Treatment and Prognosis

The treatment of both variants of rhabdomyoma consists of local surgical excision. Recurrence is uncommon but has been reported in a few cases.

Leiomyosarcoma

The leiomyosarcoma is a malignant neoplasm of smooth muscle origin, which accounts for 7% of all soft tissue sarcomas. The most common sites are the uterine wall and gastrointestinal tract. Leiomyosarcomas of the oral cavity are rare.

Clinical Features

In general leiomyosarcomas are most common in middle-aged and older adults. However, tumors in the oral and maxillofacial region occur over a wide age range without a predilection for any age group. They have been reported at various sites, but half of all oral cases occur in the jawbones. The clinical appearance is nonspecific, there is usually an enlarging mass that may or may not be painful. Secondary ulceration of the mucosal surface may occur.

Histopathologic Features

The microscopic examination of a leiomyosarcoma shows fascicles of spindle shaped cells with abundant eosinophilic cytoplasm and blunt ended, cigar shaped nuclei. Some tumors may be composed primarily of rounded epithelioid cells that have either eosinophilic or clear cytoplasm (epithelioid leiomyo sarcoma). The degree of pleomorphism varies from one tumor to the next, but smooth muscle tumors with the presence of five or more mitoses per ten high power fields should be considered malignant.

Treatment and Prognosis

The treatment of leiomyosarcoma primarily consists of radical surgical excision. Sometimes with adjunctive chemotherapy or radiation therapy.

Metastases to the Oral Soft Tissues

Metastatic tumors to the oral cavity are uncommon and represent approximately 1% of all oral malignancies. Such metastases can occur to bone or to the oral soft tissues. The mechanism by which tumors can spread to the oral cavity is poorly understood. Primary malignancies from immediately adjacent tissues might be able to spread by a lymphatic route; however, such a mechanism cannot explain metastases from tumors from lower parts of the body, which are almost certainly blood borne and should be filtered out by the lungs. One possible explanation for blood-borne metastases to the head and neck, especially in the absence of pulmonary metastases is Batson's plexus a valve less vertebral venous plexus that might allow retrograde spread of tumor cells, by passing filtration through the lungs.

Clinical Features

The most common site for oral soft tissue metastases is the gingiva, which accounts for slightly more than 50% of all cases. This is followed by the tongue, which is the site for 25% of cases. The lesion usually appears as a nodular mass that often resembles a hyperplastic or reactive growth, such as a pyogenic granuloma. Occasionally, the lesion appears as a surface ulceration, adjacent teeth may become loosened by an underlying destruction of the alveolar bone.

The presence of teeth may play an important role in the preference of metastases for the gingiva. Once malignant cells reach the oral cavity, the rich vascular network of inflamed gingival tissues may serve as a fertile site for further growth. Oral soft tissue metastases are more common in males and are seen most frequently in middle-aged and older adults. Almost any malignancy from anybody site is capable of metastasis to the oral cavity, and a wide *variety* of tumors have been reported to spread to the mouth. In the cases reported, lung cancer is responsible for more than one third of all oral soft tissue metastases in men, followed by renal carcinoma and melanoma. Although prostate cancer is common in men, metastases from these tumors have an affinity for bone and rarely occur in soft tissues. For women, breast cancer accounts for 25% of all cases, followed by malignancies of the genital organs, lung, bone, and kidney. It is probable that in the future we will see an increased number of metastatic lung cancers in women. In most cases, the primary tumor already is known when the metastatic lesion is discovered. In some cases, however, the oral lesion is the first sign of the malignant disease.

Treatment and Prognosis

The prognosis for patients with metastatic tumors is generally poor because other metastatic sites also are frequently present. Management of the oral lesion is usually palliative and should be coordinated with the patient's overall treatment.

Salivary Glands Tumors

Benign Tumors of the Salivary Glands

Oncocytoma (Oxyphilic Adenoma)

The oncocytoma is a benign salivary gland tumor composed of large epithelial cells known as oncocytes. It is a rare neoplasm, representing approximately 1% of all salivary tumors.

Clinical Features

The oncocytoma is predominantly a tumor of older adults, with a peak prevalence in the eighth decade of life. A slight female predilection has been observed but may not be significant. Oncocytomas occur primarily in the major salivary glands, especially the parotid gland. Oncocytomas of the minor salivary glands are exceedingly rare. The tumor appears as a firm, slowly growing, painless mass that rarely exceeds 4 cm in diameter. Parotid oncocytomas usually are found in the superficial lobe and are clinically indistinguishable from other benign tumors. On occasion, bilateral tumors can occur, although these may represent examples of multinodular oncocytic hyperplasia (oncocytosis).

Treatment and Prognosis

Oncocytomas are best treated by surgical excision. The prognosis after removal is good, with a low rate of recurrence. However, oncocytomas of the sinonasal glands can be locally aggressive and have been considered to be low-grade malignancies. Rare examples of histopathologically malignant oncocytomas (oncocytic carcinoma) also have been reported. These carcinomas have a relatively poor prognosis.

Oncocytosis (Nodular Oncocytic Hyperplasia)

Oncocytic metaplasia is the transformation of ductal and acinar cells to oncocytes. Such cells are uncommon before the age of 50; however, as people get older, Occasional oncocytes are a common finding in the salivary glands. Focal oncocytic metaplasia also may be a feature of other salivary gland tumors. Oncocytosis refers to both the proliferation and accumulation of oncocytes within salivary gland tissue. It may mimic a tumor, both clinically and microscopically, but it also is considered to be a metaplastic process rather than a neoplastic one.

Clinical Features

Oncocytosis is found primarily in the parotid gland; however, in rare instances, it may involve the submandibular or minor salivary glands. It can be an incidental finding in otherwise normal salivary gland tissue, but it may be extensive enough to produce clinical swelling. Usually the proliferation is multifocal and nodular, but sometimes the entire gland can be replaced by oncocytes. As with other oncocytic proliferations, oncocytosis occurs most frequently in older adults.

Treatment and Prognosis

Oncocytosis is a benign condition and often is discovered only as an incidental finding. No further treatment is necessary, and the prognosis is excellent.

Cystadenoma

Cystadenoma of the salivary glands are benign neoplasms in which the epithelium demonstrates adenomatous proliferation that is characterized by formation of multiple cystic structures. Several morphologic variants of cystadenoma have been described, of which papillary cystadenoma and mucinous cystadenoma are important.

Clinical Features

Cystadenoma is widely distributed among major and minor salivary glands. Most of the minor salivary gland tumors are seen in lips, buccal mucosa, palate and the tonsillar area. This is more common in females than males (2:1) and occurs in older age, most common in the eight decade of life. Clinically it presents as a slow growing painless slightly compressible swelling. Some of the nodules are clinically similar to mucocele.

Treatment and Prognosis

A conservative surgical procedure ensures complete removal

Warthin Tumor (Papillary Cystadenoma Lymphomatosum)

Warthin tumor is a benign neoplasm that occurs almost exclusively in the parotid gland. Although it is much less common than the pleomorphic adenoma, it represents the second most common benign parotid tumor. The name adenolymphoma also has been used for this tumor, but this term should be avoided because it overemphasizes the lymphoid component and may give the mistaken impression that the lesion is a type of lymphoma. The pathogenesis of these tumors is uncertain. The traditional hypothesis suggests that they arise from heterotopic salivary gland tissue found within parotid lymphnodes. However, it also has been suggested that these tumors may develop from a proliferation of salivary gland ductal epithelium that is associated with secondary formation of lymphoid tissue. A number of studies have demonstrated a strong association between the development of this tumor and smoking. Smokers have an eight fold greater risk for Warthin tumor than do nonsmokers. Epstein-Barr virus also has been implicated in the pathogenesis of Warthin tumor.

Clinical Features

The Warthin tumor usually appears as a slowly growing, painless, nodular mass of the parotid gland. It may be firm or fluctuant to palpation. The tumor most frequently occurs in the tail of the parotid near the angle of the mandible, and it may be noted for many months before the patient seeks a diagnosis. One unique feature is the tendency of Warthin tumor to occur bilaterally. Most of these bilateral tumors do not occur simultaneously but are metachronous (occurring at different times). In rare instances, the Warthin tumor has been reported within the submandibular gland or minor salivary glands. However, because the lymphoid component is often less pronounced in these extraparotid sites, the pathologist should exercise caution to avoid over diagnosis of a lesion.

Warthin tumor most often occurs in older adults, with a peak prevalence in the sixth and seventh decades of life. Most studies show a decided male predilection, with some early studies demonstrating a male-to-female ratio up to 10 to 1. However, more recent investigations show a more balanced sex ratio, because Warthin tumors have been associated with cigarette smoking. This changing sex ratio may be are flection of the increased prevalence of smoking in females over the past few decades.

Treatment and Prognosis

Surgical removal is the treatment of choice for patients with Warthin tumor. The procedure usually is easily accomplished because of the superficial location of the tumor.

Canalicular Adenoma

The canalicular adenoma is an uncommon tumor that occurs almost exclusively in the minor salivary glands. Because of its uniform microscopic pattern, the canalicular adenoma also has been called a "monomorphic adenoma." However, because this term also has been applied to other tumors, its use probably should be discontinued.

Clinical Features

The canalicular adenoma shows a striking predilection for the upper lip, with nearly 75% occurring in this location. It represents the first or second most common tumor (along with pleomorphic adenoma) of the upper lip. The buccal mucosa is the second most common site. Occurrence in other minor salivary glands is uncommon and canalicular adenomas of the parotid gland are rare. The tumor nearly always occurs in older adults, with a peak prevalence in the seventh decade of life. There is a definite female predominance, ranging from 1.2 to 1.8 females for each male. The canalicular adenoma appears as a slowly growing, painless mass that usually ranges from several millimeters to 2 cm. It may be firm or somewhat fluctuant to palpation. The overlying mucosa may be normal in color or bluish and can be mistaken for a mucocele. However, mucoceles of the upper lip are rare. In some instances the lesion has been noted to be multifocal, with multiple separate tumors discovered in the upper lip or buccal mucosa.

Treatment and Prognosis

The canalicular adenoma is best treated by local surgical excision. Recurrence is uncommon and actually may represent cases that are multifocal in nature.

Basal Cell Adenoma

The basal cell adenoma is a benign salivary tumor that derives its name from the basaloid appearance of the tumor cells. It is an uncommon neoplasm that represents only 1 to 2% of all salivary tumors. Because of its uniform histopathologic appearance. It often has been classified as one of the monomorphic adenomas.

Clinical Features

Unlike then canalicular adenoma, the basal cell adenoma is primarily a tumor of the parotid gland, with around 75% of all cases occurring there. However, the minor glands represent the second most common site, specifically the glands of the upper lip and buccal mucosa. The tumor can occur at any age but is most common in middle aged and older adults, with a peak prevalence in the seventh decade of life. The tumor appears to be more common in females, with some studies showing as high as a 2: 1 female to male ratio. Clinically the basal cell adenoma appears as a slowly growing freely movable mass similar to a pleomorphic adenoma. Most tumors are less than 3 cm in diameter. Parotid tumors usually are located within the superficial lobe of the gland.

One subtype, the membranous basal cell adenoma, appears to be hereditary, often occurring in combination with skin appendage tumors, such as dermal cylindromas and trichoepitheliomas. Multiple bilateral tumors may develop within the parotids. Because these tumors often bear a histopathologic resemblance to the skin tumors, they also have been called dermal analogue tumors.

Treatment and Prognosis

The treatment of basal cell adenoma is similar to that of pleomorphic adenoma and consists of complete surgical removal. Recurrence is rare for most histopathologic subtypes.

Ductal Papillomas (Sialadenoma Papilliferum; Intraductal Papilloma and Inverted Ductal Papilloma)

A number of salivary gland tumors can be characterized microscopically by a papillomatous pattern. The sialadenoma papilliferum, intraductal papilloma, and inverted ductal papilloma are three rare salivary tumors that also show unique papillomatous features.

Clinical Features

The sialadenoma papilliferum most commonly arises from the minor salivary glands, especially on the palate, although it also has been reported in the parotid gland. It usually is seen in older adults and has a 1.5: 1 male to female ratio. The tumor appears as an exophytic, papillary surface growth that is clinically similar to the common squamous papilloma. The intraductal papilloma is an ill defined lesion that often has been confused with other salivary gland lesions, such as the papillary cystadenoma. It usually occurs in adults and is most common in the minor salivary glands, where it appears as a submucosal swelling. The inverted ductal papilloma is a rare tumor that has been described only in the minor salivary glands of adults. The lower lip and mandibular vestibule are the most common locations. The lesion usually appears as an asymptomatic submucosal nodule, which sometimes may show a pit or indentation in the overlying surface mucosa.

Treatment and Prognosis

All three forms of ductal papilloma are best treated by conservative surgical excision. Recurrence is rare.

Malignant Tumors of Salivary Glands

Acinic Cell Adenocarcinoma

The acinic cell adenocarcinoma is a salivary gland malignancy with cells that show serous acinar differentiation. Because many of these tumors act in a nonaggressive fashion and are associated with a good prognosis. This neoplasm formerly was called acinic cell tumor, a nonspecific designation that did not indicate whether the lesion was benign or malignant. However, because some of these tumors do metastasize or recur and cause death, it is generally agreed today that acinic cell adenocarcinoma should be considered a low-grade malignancy.

Clinical Features

Around 85% of all acinic cell adenocarcinomas occur in the parotid gland. A logical finding because this is the largest gland and one that is composed entirely of serous elements. It is much less common in the submandibular gland. The tumor occurs over a broad age range, with a relatively even peak prevalence stretching from the second to the seventh decades of life. The tumor usually appears as a slowly growing mass and the lesion often is appears for many months or years before a diagnosis is made. The tumor may be otherwise asymptomatic, although associated pain or tenderness sometimes are reported. Facial nerve paralysis is an infrequent but ominous sign for parotid tumors.

Histopathologic Features

Acinic cell adenocarcinomas are highly variable in their microscopic appearance. The tumor often is well circumscribed and sometimes may even appear encapsulated; however some tumors exhibit an infiltrative growth pattern. The most characteristic cell is one with features of the serous acinar cell, with abundant granular basophilic cytoplasm and a round, darkly stained eccentric nucleus. These cells are fairly uniform in appearance and mitotic activity is uncommon. Other cells may resemble intercalated duct cells and some tumors also have cells with a clear, vacuolated cytoplasm. Several growth patterns may be seen. The solid variety consists of numerous well-differentiated acinar cells arranged in a pattern that resembles normal parotid gland tissue, in the microcystic variety. Multiple small cystic spaces are created that may contain some mucinous or eosinophilic material. In the papillary-cystic variety, larger cystic areas are formed that are lined by epithelium having papillary projections into the cystic spaces. The follicular variety has an appearance similar to that of thyroid tissue. A lymphoid infiltrate is not unusual, sometimes with germinal center formation, is not unusual.

Treatment and Prognosis

Acinic cell adenocarcinomas confined to the superficial lobe of the parotid gland are best treated by lobectomy; for those in the deep lobe, total parotidectomy is usually necessary. The facial nerve may need to be sacrificed if it is involved by tumor. Submandibular tumors are managed by total removal of the gland and minor gland tumors are treated with assured surgical excision. Lymph node dissection is not indicated unless there is clinical evidence of metastatic disease. Adjunctive radiation therapy may be considered for uncontrolled local disease.

Carcinoma Ex Pleomorphic Adenoma; Ex Mixed Tumor; Carcinosarcoma and Metastasizing Mixed Tumor

Malignant mixed tumors represent malignant counterparts to the benign mixed tumor pleomorphic adenoma. These uncommon neoplasms can be divided into three categories:

1. Carcinoma ex pleomorphic adenoma ex mixed tumor
2. Carcinosarcoma
3. Metastasizing mixed tumor

The most common of these is the carcinoma ex pleomorphic adenoma, which is characterized by malignant transformation of the epithelial component of a previously benign pleomorphic adenoma. The carcinosarcoma is a rare "mixed" tumor in which both carcinomatous and sarcomatous elements are present. The metastasizing mixed tumor has histopathologic features that are identical to the common pleomorphic adenoma (mixed tumor). In spite of its benign appearance, however, the lesion metastasizes. The metastatic tumor also has a benign microscopic appearance, usually similar to that of the primary lesion.

Clinical Features

Carcinoma ex pleomorphic adenoma: There is fairly convincing evidence that the carcinoma ex pleomorphic adenoma represents a malignant transformation with in what was previously a benign neoplasm. It is most common in middle-aged and older adults. With a peak prevalence in the sixth to eighth decades of life. In addition, patients may report that a mass has been present for many years, sometimes undergoing a recent rapid growth with associated pain or ulceration. However, some tumors may have a short duration. Over 80% of cases of carcinoma ex pleomorphic adenoma are seen within the major glands, primarily the parotid gland. Nearly two thirds of minor salivary gland cases occur on the palate. There is a slight female predilection. Although pain or recent rapid grow this not unusual. Many cases present as a painless mass that is indistinguishable from a benign tumor. Parotid tumors may produce facial nerve palsy.

Carcinosarcoma: The carcinosarcoma is an extremely rare tumor. Most cases have been reported in the parotid gland, but the lesion also has been seen in the submandibular gland and minor salivary glands. The clinical signs and symptoms are similar to those of the carcinoma ex pleomorphic adenoma. Some patients have a previous history of a benign pleomorphic adenoma.

Metastasizing mixed tumor: The metastasizing mixed tumor is also quite rare. As with other malignant mixed tumors, most cases originate in the parotid gland, but the primary tumor also may occur in the submandibular gland or minor salivary glands. Metastases have been found most frequently in the bones or lung, but they also can occur in other sites. Such as regional lymph nodes or the liver. Most patients have a history of a benign mixed tumor, which may have been excised many years earlier. Many times the primary tumor exhibits multiple recurrences before metastasis occurs.

Treatment and Prognosis

Carcinoma ex pleomorphic adenoma: Invasive carcinoma ex pleomorphic adenoma usually is best treated by wide excision, possibly in conjunction with local lymph node dissection and adjunctive radiation therapy.

Carcinosarcoma: Carcinosarcomas are treated by radical surgical excision, which may be combined with radiation therapy and chemotherapy. The prognosis is poor.

Metastasizing mixed tumor: The treatment for a metastasizing mixed tumor consists of surgical excision of both the primary tumor and metastatic sites.

Adenoid Cystic Carcinoma

The adenoid cystic carcinoma is one of the more common and best recognized salivary malignancies. Because of its distinctive histopathologic features.

Clinical and Radiographic Features

The adenoid cystic carcinoma can occur in any salivary gland site, but approximately develop within the minor salivary glands. The palate is the most common site for minor gland tumors. The remaining tumors are found mostly in the parotid and submandibular glands, with a fairly even distribution between these two sites. On an individual basis, however, a striking difference can be seen among the various glands. The lesion is most common in middle-aged adults. There is a fairly equal sex distribution, although some studies have shown a slight female predilection.

The adenoid cystic carcinoma usually appears as a slowly growing mass. Pain is a common and important finding, occasionally occurring early in the course of the disease before there is a noticeable swelling. Patients often complain of a constant, low-grade, dull ache, which gradually increases in intensity. Facial nerve paralysis may develop with parotid tumors. Palatal tumors can be smooth surfaced or ulcerated. Tumors arising in the palate or maxillary sinus may show radiographic evidence of bone destruction.

Treatment and Prognosis

Adenoid cystic carcinoma is a relentless tumor that is prone to local recurrence and eventual distant metastasis. Surgical excision is usually the treatment of choice, and adjunct radiation therapy may slightly *improve patient* survival in some cases.

Polymorphous Low-grade Adenocarcinoma (Lobular Carcinoma and Terminal Duct Carcinoma)

The polymorphous low-grade adenocarcinoma is a recently recognized type of salivary malignancy that was first described in 1983.

Clinical Features

The polymorphous low-grade adenocarcinoma is almost exclusively a tumor of the minor salivary glands. However, rare examples also have been reported in the major glands, either arising denovo or as the malignant component of a carcinoma ex pleomorphic adenoma. Sixty-five percent occur on the hard or soft palate. With the upper lip and buccal mucosa being the next most common locations. It is most common in older adults, having a peak prevalence in the sixth to eighth decades of life. Two thirds of all cases occur in females. The tumor most often appears as a pain less mass that may have been present for a long time with slow growth. Occasionally it is associated with bleeding or discomfort. Tumor can erode or infiltrate the underlying bone.

Treatment and Prognosis

The polymorphous low-grade adenocarcinoma is best treated by wide surgical excision, sometimes including resection of the underlying bone.

Mucoepidermoid Carcinoma

The mucoepidermoid carcinoma is one of the most common salivary gland malignancies. Because of its highly variable biologic potential, it was originally called mucoepidermoid tumor.

Clinical Features

The tumor occurs fairly evenly over a wide age range, extending from the second to seventh decades of life. A slight female predilection has been noted. Some tumors have been associated with a previous history of radiation therapy to the head and neck region. The mucoepidermoid carcinoma is most common in the parotid gland and usually appears as an asymptomatic swelling. Most patients are aware of the lesion for a year or less, although some report a mass of many years duration. Pain or facial nerve palsy may develop usually in association with high -grade tumors, the minor glands constitute the second most common site especially the palate. Minor gland tumors also typically appear as asymptomatic swellings. Which are sometimes fluctuant and have a blue or red color that can be mistaken clinically for a mucocele. Although the lower lip, floor of mouth, tongue and retro molar pad areas are uncommon locations for salivary gland neoplasia. The mucoepidermoid carcinoma is the most common salivary tumor in each of these sites.

Treatment and Prognosis

The treatment of mucoepidermoid carcinoma is predicated by the location, histopathologic grade, and clinical stage of the tumor. Early-stage tumors of the parotid often can be treated by subtotal parotidectomy with preservation of the facial nerve, Advanced tumors may necessitate total removal of the parotid gland, with sacrifice of the facial nerve. Submandibular gland tumors are treated by total removal of the gland. Mucoepidermoid carcinomas of the minor glands usually are treated by assured surgical excision.

Odontogenic Tumors

Ameloblastoma

The ameloblastoma is the most common clinically significant odontogenic tumor. Theoretically, they may arise from rests of dental lamina, from a developing enamel organ, from the epithelial lining of an odontogenic cyst or from the basal cells of the oral mucosa. Ameloblastomas are slow-growing, locally invasive tumors that run a benign course in most cases. They occur in three different clinic radiographic situations, which deserve separate consideration because of differing therapeutic considerations and prognosis. These are:

1. Conventional solid or multicystic
2. Unicystic
3. Peripheral (extra osseous)

Conventional Solid or Multicystic Intraosseous Ameloblastoma

Clinical and Radiographic Features

Conventional solid or multicystic intraosseous ameloblastoma is encountered in patients over a wide age range. The tumor shows an approximately equal prevalence in the third to seventh decades of life. There is no significant gender predilection. Conventional ameloblastomas occur in the mandible, most often in the molar ascending ramus area. About 15% of ameloblastomas occur in the maxilla, usually in the posterior regions. The tumor is often asymptomatic, and smaller lesions are detected only during a radiographic examination. A painless swelling or expansion of the jaw is the usual clinical presentation. If untreated, the lesion may grow slowly to massive. Pain and paresthesia are uncommon, even with large tumors. The most typical radiographic feature is that of a multilocular radiolucent lesion. The lesion is often described as having a "soap bubble" appearance when the radiolucent loculations are large and as *being* "honeycombed" when the loculations are small. Buccal and lingual cortical expansion is frequently present. Resorption of the roots of teeth adjacent to the tumor is common. In many cases, an unerupted tooth, most often a mandibular third molar is associated with the radiolucent defect. Solid ameloblastomas may radiographically appear as unilocular radiolucent defects, which may resemble almost any type of cystic lesion. The margins of these radiolucent lesion show ever, often show irregular scalloping. Although the radiographic features, particularly of the typical multilocular defect, may be highly suggestive of ameloblastoma.

Treatment and Prognosis

Patients with conventional solid or multicystic intra osseous ameloblastomas have been treated by a variety of means. These range from simple enucleation and curettage to *en bloc* resection.

Malignant Ameloblastoma and Ameloblastic Carcinoma

Rarely, an ameloblastoma exhibits frank malignant behavior with development of metastases. The frequency of malignant behavior in ameloblastomas is difficult to determine but probably occurs in far less than 1% of all ameloblastomas. The terminology for these lesions is somewhat controversial. The term malignant ameloblastoma should be used for a tumor that shows the histopathologic features of ameloblastoma. Both in the primary tumor and in the metastatic deposits. The term ameloblastic carcinoma should be reserved for an ameloblastoma that has cytologic features of malignancy in the primary tumor. In a recurrence, or in any metastatic deposit, these lesions may follow a markedly aggressive local course, but metastases do not necessarily occur.

Clinical and Radiographic Features

Malignant ameloblastomas have been observed in patients who range in age from 4 to 75 years. Metastases from ameloblastomas are most often found in the lungs. These have sometimes been regarded as aspiration or implant metastases. However, the peripheral location of some of these lung metastases suggests that they must have occurred by blood or lymphatic routes rather than aspiration. Cervical lymph nodes are the second most common site for metastasis of an ameloblastoma. Spread to vertebrae, other bones and viscera has also occasionally been confirmed. The radiographic findings of malignant ameloblastomas may be essentially the same as those in typical non metastasizing ameloblastomas. Ameloblastic carcinomas are often more aggressive lesions with ill-defined margins and cortical destruction.

Treatment and Prognosis

The prognosis of patients with malignant ameloblastomas appears to be poor.

Clear Cell Odontogenic Carcinoma (Clear Cell Odontogenic Tumor)

Clear cell odontogenic carcinoma is a rare jaw tumor that was first described in 1985. The tumor appears to be of odontogenic origin, but its histogenesis is uncertain. Histochemical and ultrastructural studies show that the clear cells, which are the prominent feature of this neoplasm, have similarities to glycogen rich presecretory ameloblasts.

Clinical and Radiographic Features

Because of the paucity of reported cases, there is little valid clinical information regarding the clear cell odontogenic carcinoma. Most cases are diagnosed in patients older than age 50, and both the mandible and maxilla have been involved. Some patients complain of pain and bony swelling; others are relatively symptom- free. Radiographically, the lesions appear as unilocular or multilocular radiolucencies. The margins of the radiolucency are often somewhat ill defined or irregular.

Treatment and Prognosis

Clear cell odontogenic carcinomas largely demonstrate an aggressive clinical course, with invasion of contiguous structures and a tendency to recur. Most patients require fairly radical surgery. Pulmonary or lymphatic metastases may occur.

Squamous Odontogenic Tumor

Squamous odontogenic tumor is a rare benign odontogenic neoplasm that was first described in 1975 and is now recognized as a distinct entity. Most of these have been located within bone, although a few peripheral examples have been described. The squamous odontogenic tumor may arise from neoplastic transformation of dental lamina rests or perhaps the epithelial rests of Malassez. The tumor appears to originate within the periodontal ligament that is associated with the lateral root surface of an erupted tooth.

Clinical and Radiographic Features

Squamous odontogenic tumors have been found in patients whose ages ranged from 8 to 74 years. They are randomly distributed throughout the alveolar processes of the maxilla and mandible, with no site of predilection. A few patients have had multiple squamous odontogenic tumors that involved several quadrants of the mouth. There is no apparent sex predilection. A painless or mildly painful gingival swelling, often associated with mobility of the associated teeth, is the most common complaint. About 25% of reported patients have had no symptoms, and their lesions were detected during a radiographic examination. The radiographic findings are not specific or diagnostic and consist of a triangular radiolucent defect lateral to the root or roots of the teeth. In some instances, this suggests vertical periodontal bone loss. The radiolucent area may be somewhat ill defined or may show a well defined sclerotic margin. Most examples are relatively small lesions that seldom exceed 1.5 cm in greatest diameter.

Treatment and Prognosis

Conservative local excision or curettage appears to be effective for patients with squamous odontogenic tumors, and most reported cases have not recurred after local excision. A few instances of recurrence have been reported

Tumors of Odontogenic Ectomesenchyme

Central Odontogenic Fibroma

The central odontogenic fibroma is an uncommon and somewhat controversial lesion. Formerly, some oral and maxillofacial pathologists designated solid fibrous masses that were almost always associated with the crown of an unerupted tooth as odontogenic fibromas. Most oral and maxillofacial pathologists today consider such lesions to represent only hyperplastic dental follicles, and these should not be considered to be neoplasms.

Clinical and Radiographic Features

Odontogenic fibromas have been reported in patients whose ages ranged from 4 to 80 years, of those cases reported in the literature, a 2.2 to 1 female predilection has been noted. About 45% of reported cases have occurred in the maxilla; most maxillary lesions are located anterior to the first molar tooth. In the mandible, however, about half of the tumors are located posterior to the first molar. One third of odontogenic fibromas are associated with an unerupted tooth. Smaller odontogenic fibromas are usually completely asymptomatic; larger lesions may be associated with localized bony expansion or loosening of teeth.

Radiographically, smaller odontogenic fibromas tend to be well-defined, unilocular, radiolucent lesions often associated with the periradicular area of erupted teeth. Larger lesions tend to be multilocular radiolucencies. Many lesions have a sclerotic border. Root resorption of associated teeth is common, and lesions located between the teeth often cause root divergence. Approximately 12% of central odontogenic fibromas will exhibit radiopaque flecks within the lesion.

Treatment and Prognosis

Odontogenic fibromas are usually treated by enucleation and vigorous curettage. Although the tumor does not have a definite capsule, it appears to have a limited growth potential, particularly in the anterior regions of the jaws. A few recurrences have been documented, but the prognosis is very good.

Peripheral Odontogenic Fibroma

The relatively uncommon peripheral odontogenic fibroma is considered to represent the soft tissue counterpart of the central (lntraosseous) odontogenic fibroma.

Clinical and Radiographic Features

The peripheral odontogenic fibroma appears as a firm, slow-growing, and usually sessile gingival mass covered by normal-appearing mucosa. Rarely, multifocal or diffuse lesions have been described. Clinically, the peripheral odontogenic fibroma cannot be distinguished from the much more common fibrous gingival lesions. The lesion is most often encountered on the facial gingiva of the mandible. Most lesions are between 0.5 and 1.5 cm in diameter and they infrequently cause displacement of the teeth. Peripheral odontogenic fibroma as have been recorded in patients over a wide age range, with most identified from the second to the seventh decades of life.

Radiographic studies demonstrate a soft tissue mass, which in some cases has shown areas of calcification. The lesion, however, does not involve the underlying bone.

Treatment and Prognosis

The peripheral odontogenic fibroma is treated by local surgical excision, and the prognosis is excellent. Recurrence of this lesion has been documented.

Granular Cell Odontogenic Tumor (Granular Cell Odontogenic Fibroma)

The rare granular cell odontogenic tumor was initially reported as "granular cell ameloblastic fibroma". Subsequently, it was designated as granular cell odontogenic fibroma, but the noncommittal term granular cell odontogenic tumor is probably more appropriate, given the controversial nature of the lesion.

Clinical and Radiographic Features

Patients with granular cell odontogenic tumors have all been adults at the time of diagnosis, with over half being older than 40 years of age. The tumor occurs primarily in the mandible and most often in the premolar and molar region. Some lesions are completely asymptomatic; others present as a painless, localized expansion of the affected area.

Radiographically, the lesion appears as a well demarcated radiolucency, which may be unilocular or multilocular and occasionally shows small calcifications.

Treatment and Prognosis

The granular cell odontogenic fibroma appears to be completely benign and responds well to curettage. No recurrences have been reported.

MEDICAL EMERGENCIES

In dental practice medical emergency situations are expected especially while treating geriatric population. Hence a dental clinic should be equipped with emergency drugs. The commonest emergencies seen are syncope, hypoglycaemia, asthma, anaphylaxis, angina and seizures.

Emergency drugs

- Oxygen (inhalation)
- Glyceryl trinitrate (GTN) (sublingual)
- Aspirin (dispersible)
- Salbutamol aerosol inhaler
- Adrenaline injection (intramuscular)
- Glucagon injection (intramuscular/subcutaneous)
- Oral glucose solution (oral)
- Midazolam (buccal sulcus/inhalation)

The drugs should be checked for expiry date and maintained regularly.

ABCDE approach to an emergency patient

An abnormal patient colour, pulse rate or breathing can signal some impending emergencies.

A – Airway

B – Breathing

C – Circulation

D – Disability

E – Exposure (to facilitate placement of AED paddles) or exposing parts to be examined.

Airway

A head tilt, chin lift or jaw thrust (avoids cervical spine extension) will open the airway. Any visible foreign bodies, blood or debris should be removed. Clearing the mouth should be done with great care and avoid pushing material into upper airway. 'Finger sweep' is best in adults. Airway adjuncts such as oropharyngeal airway can be used if patient is unconscious. Administration of oxygen is also important. Patients with chronic obstructive pulmonary disease retain carbondioxide and should be given high concentration of oxygen.

Breathing

The clinician should look for chest movements, listen for breath sounds at patient's mouth and feel for air on the rescuer's cheek with the rescuer's head turned against patient's mouth. This should be done within 10 seconds and breathing should be determined. If breathing is not normal cardiopulmonary resuscitation (CPR) should be commenced. Patient may breath barely or gasp in the first few minutes after cardiac arrest and it should not be mistaken for normal breathing – ' Agonal gasps'.

If patient is not breathing normally:

- Start chest compressions.
- Place the heel of one hand in the centre of patient's chest and other hand on top of the first hand.
- Interlock the fingers.

- Rescuer should be present vertically above the patient's chest. With straight arms, sternum should be depressed 4 – 5 cm (Pressure should not be applied over the ribs, upper abdomen or lower end of the sternum).
- The pressure should be released after each compression so that the rib cage recoils to its rest position, but the hands should be maintained in contact with the sternum.
- The rate should be approximately 100 times per minute.
- After 30 compressions, airway should be opened using head tilt and chin lift and two rescue breaths should be given.
- Rescue breaths are carried out using bag and mask or mouth to mouth (with nostrils closed between thumb and index finger) or mouth to mask.

Circulation

- Most common cause of a collapse of circulatory origin is the simple faint (vasovagal syncope)
- If the patient is laid flat with legs raised rapid recovery occurs.
- If recovery does not occur other causes than a faint must be considered.
- Checking the carotid pulse to diagnose cardiac arrest can be unreliable and checking the carotid pulse should be carried out only by those who are proficient in doing this.
- Identification of agonal gasps as a sign to commence CPR are highlighted.

Disability

- Disability is assessment of neurological status of the patient.
- It refers to level of consciousness
- Hypoxia or hypercapnia (increased blood level of carbon dioxide) are possible causes, together with certain sedative or analgesic drugs.
- Hypoxia or hypertension should be excluded and attention to the airway, giving supplemental oxygen and supporting patient's circulation (by lying them supine and raising their legs).

- Unconscious patients who are breathing and have a pulse should be placed in recovery position if they are unable to maintain their own airway.

Exposure

Exposure is loosening or removal of some of the patient's clothes for application of defibrillator paddles or for examination purposes if the patient has been involved in a traumatic incident.

Defibrillation

Defibrillation is the term used to describe controlled electrical shock administered to the fibrillating heart, which may restore an organized rhythm enabling the heart to contract effectively. Early defibrillation in cardiac arrest is important. Ventricular fibrillation is the most common cause of cardiac arrest. It is a rapid and chaotic rhythm and as result the heart is unable to contract effectively and unable to sustain its function as a pump. The only effective treatment for ventricular fibrillation is defibrillation.

The provision of defibrillation has been made easier by development of automated external defibrillators (AEDS).

The device analyses the victim's heart rhythm, determines the need for a shock and then delivers it if advised. CPR should not be interrupted or delayed to set up an AED.

The AED pads placement requires practical training and experience. One pad placed to the right of the sternum below the clavicle. The other pad should be placed in the left side mid-axillary line, central on the fifth intercostals space. This electrode works best if orientated vertically. This position should be clear of any breast tissue.

Vasovagal Syncope

Vasovagal syncope or a simple faint is loss of consciousness due to inadequate cerebral perfusion. It is a reflex mediated by autonomic nerves leading to widespread vasodilatation in the splanchnic and skeletal vessels and bradycardia resulting in diminished cerebral perfusion. Fainting can be precipitated by pain or emotional stress, changes in posture or hypoxia.

Patient feels faint/dizzy, pallor, sweating, pulse rate slows, low blood pressure, nausea and/or vomiting, loss of consciousness.

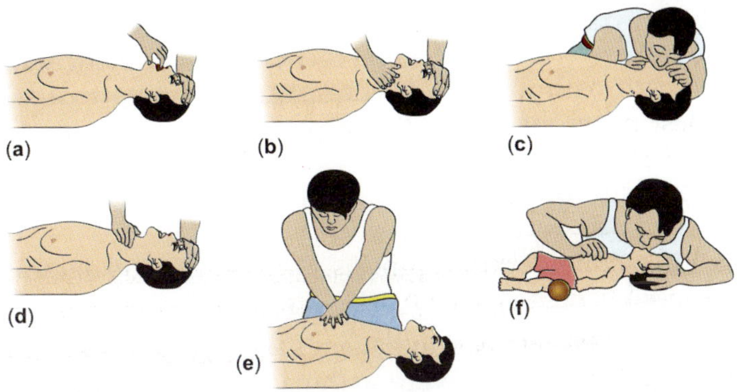

Figs 6.9A to F: (a) Finger sweep of foreign body; (b) head tilt chin lift; (c) mouth to mouth breathing; (d) checking the pulse; (e) chest compressions; and (f) CPR in a child

Lie the patient flat and raise their legs and patient airway must be maintained. If recovery is delayed, oxygen should be administered and other causes of loss of consciousness be considered.

Hyperventilation

Anxiety is the principal precipitating factor, symptoms are anxiety, dizziness, lightheadedness, weakness, paresthesia, tetany, chest pain/palpitation, breathlessness.

Exclude other causes for symptoms before diagnosing hyperventilation. Make the patient to rebreath their own exhaled air to increase the amount of inhaled carboindioxide – a paper bag placed over nose and mouth. Patient's cupped hands would be alternative but less satisfactory.

Hyperventilation leads to carbondioxide being washed out of the body, producing an alkalosis. If hyperventilation persists, carpal and pedal spasm may be seen. Rebreathing exhaled air helps to return situation normal.

Asthma

Severe asthma is potential life-threatening condition and attack may be precipitated by exertion, anxiety, infection of exposure to an allergen. It is important that asthmatic patients bring their usual inhaler with them – if they have not brought their inhaler, then unless there is one in the emergency kit, treatment should be deferred. If asthma is in severe phase, elective treatment may be best postponed. NSAIDs may worsen asthma and are therefore best avoided.

Symptoms are breathlessness, expiratory wheezing, use of accessory muscles of respiration and tachycardia.

In life-threatening asthma cyanosis, bradycardia and decreased level of consciousness are seen

Most attacks will respond to patient's own inhaler. If no rapid response, or features of severe asthma call an ambulance. A medical assessment should be arranged for patients who require additional doses of bronchodilator to end an attack. If patients show any of the signs of life-threatening asthma, urgent medical assessment should be arranged. Ten litres of oxygen per minute should be given while awaiting transfer. Four to six actuations from the salbutamol inhaler via a spacer device should be used and repeated every 10 minutes.

Chest Pain (Cardiac Origin)

Patients with previous history of cardiac disease mostly suffer chest pain from a cardiac origin in dental surgery. Medication used by patient to control angina should be brought or it should be readily to hand in the emergency kit.

Pain of angina is described as a crushing or band-like tightness of the chest which may radiate to left arm or mandible. The pain of myocardial infarction will be similar to that of angina, but more severe and unlike angina, will not be relieved by glyceryl trinitrate (GTN). In case of angina, the patient should use their GTN spray, usually relieve the symptoms.

Sign and Symptoms of Myocardial Infarction

- Severe crushing chest pain, which may radiate to the shoulders and down arms and into the mandible.
- The skin becomes pale and clammy.
- Shortness of breath
- Pulse becomes weak and patient becomes hypotensive.
- Nausea and vomiting

To treat myocardial infarction practitioner should remain calm, and call for help immediately. Most patients are best managed in sitting position and patients who feel faint should be laid flat. High flow oxygen and sublingual GTN spray can be given. A patient who had a surgical dental treatment should be highlighted since use of thrombolytic therapy may lead to significant risk of hemorrhage. If patient becomes unresponsive, the clinician should check for signs of life and start CPR if necessary.

Epilepsy

Medical history reveals that the patient has epilepsy and the natures of seizures, frequency and degree of control should be enquired. Type of medication and its efficacy should be determined.

Symptoms

- Patients may have and 'aura' that a seizure is going to happen.
- Tonic phase—loss of consciousness, patient becomes rigid, falls and becomes cyanosed.
- Clonic phase—jerking movements of limbs, tongue may be bitten.
- Frothing at the mouth, urinary incontinence.
- Seizure gradually abates few minutes but patient may remain unconscious may be confused after regaining consciousness.
- Hypoglycemia may present as a fit and should be borne in mind—blood glucose measurement at an early is therefore wise.

The decision to give medication should be made if seizures are prolonged. If possible, high flow oxygen should be administered. The possibility of the patient's airway becoming occluded should be constantly remembered and the airway must be protected.

Midazolam given through the buccal or intranasal route(10 mg for adults)

For children

1 to 5 years (5 mg)

5 to 10 years (7.5 mg)

Greater than 10 years (10 mg)

Patients with poorly controlled epilepsy (parents of some children) will carry rectal diazepam. In the absence of rapid response to treatment, call an ambulance.

Diabetic Emergencies

A history of recurrent hypoglycaemic episodes and markedly varying blood glucose levels (from the patient's measurement) suggest that a patient attending for treatment is more likely to develop hypoglycaemia. Ensure that diabetic patients have had their normal medication and something to eat prior to attending.

Hypoglycaemia shows trembling, hunger, sweating, headache and slurring of speech, pins and needles in lips and tongue, seizures and unconsciousness. Hypoglycaemia can treated by:

- Lay patient flat
- If patient is conscious give oral glucose
- If unconscious give glucagons intramuscularly
- Get medical help
- If patient not responding to glucagons or those who have exhausted their supplies of liver glycogen, 20 ml of intravenous glucose solution is given. It takes 5–10 minutes to the effective.
- Once the patients regains consciousness and has an intact gag reflex – orally glucose should be given.

Principle of treatment of hyperglycaemia is through intravenous rehydration.

Allergies

Anaphylaxis: Type I hypersensitivity reaction (Ig E involved). Free antigen binds to IgE leads to release of vasoactive peptides and histamine.

Penicillin and latex are most likely causes in oral surgery. Local anaesthetics are rarely responsible.

Rashes, erythema, flushing/pallor, laryngeal edema, bronchospasm leading to stridor, wheezing and hoarseness, respiratory arrest leading to cardiac arrest, vasodilation leading to low blood pressure and collapse are the symptoms.

ABCDE approach should be used. Manage airway and breathing by administering oxygen. Blood pressure restored by lying patient flat and raising their legs.

Adrenaline administered in life threatening anaphylaxis (0.5 ml of 1 in 1000 adrenaline intramuscular). Site for injection is anterolateral mid-third of thigh but deltoid muscle may be used.

Only drug required to be administered by dental practitioners is adrenaline.

Angioedema: Angioedema is triggered when mast cells release histamine and other chemicals into the blood, producing rapid swelling, which may life-threatening if the airway is involved. It may be precipitated by latex and penicillin. Hereditary angioneurotic edema is caused by complement activation resulting from deficiency of inhibitor enzyme C1 esterase. C1 esterase inhibitor concentrates are available to supplement deficiency. Such supplements should be administered prior to surgical treatment.

Choking and Aspiration

Patient suspected with aspirated foreign body, they should be allowed to cough vigorously to clear airway and cough up the object. An inhaled foreign body may lead to either mild or severe airway obstruction.

Back blows should be delivered by standing to the side of the patient and slightly behind. The chest should be supported with one hand and the victim leant well forwards so that when the obstruction is dislodged it is expelled from the mouth rather than passing further down the airway. Five sharp blows should be given between shoulder blades with the heel of other hand.

After each back blow check for obstruction relief, if back blow fails, abdominal thrusts should be given.

- Stand behind the victim and put both arms around the upper part of the abdomen and lean then forwards.
- Rescuer's fist clenched and placed between the umbilicus and lower end of sternum.
- Clenched fist gasped with other hand and pulled sharply inwards and outwards.
- Repeat 5 times
- Back blows and abdominal thrusts continued in a cyclical fashion.

If foreign body has been inhaled, refer with chest X-ray. Bronchoscopy or even thoracotomy may be needed to retrieve it.

Adrenal Insufficiency

It would happen as result of dental treatment and it is rare.

Symptoms include loss of consciousness, rapid weak or impalpable pulse and blood pressure falls rapidly. History of recently used or currently used corticosteroids should be enquired. Acute adrenal insufficiency can be presented by the administration of a steroid boost prior to treatment. Cover comprises 10 mg hydrocortisone administered intramuscularly or intravenously. Patients systemically unwell are also recommended to have a prophylactic increase in steroid dose.

Patients with Addison's disease is to double the patient's steroid dose before significant dental treatment under local anaesthesia and continue for 24 hours.

Lay the patient flat and raise their legs. Ensure clear airway and administer oxygen. If competent give 200 mg hydrocortisone intravenously.

Stroke

Stroke may be haemorrhagic or embolic but clinically the effects are same. There may be loss of consciousness and weakness of limbs on one side. As stroke causes an upper motor neurone lesion the forehead muscles of facial expression will be unaffected. Speech may become slurred.

Airway should be maintained and medical review arranged. High flow is oxygen given.

Local Anaesthetic Emergencies

Allergy to local anaesthetic is rare but should be managed as any other case of anaphylaxis. The signs and symptoms in allergy are those of anaphylaxis.

Fainting in association with the injection of local anaesthetic is more common and be avoided by administering local anaesthetic while in supine position.

Medical emergencies can occur at any time and surgeon must be proficient at diagnosing them and giving initial management.

BIBLIOGRAPHY

1. Orban's Oral Histology and Embryology; G.S.Kumar, 12th edition, 2006.
2. Tencate's Oral histology development, structure and function, 6th edition.
3. A Textbook of Geriatrics and Gerontology; OP Sharma, 2004.
4. Shafer's Textbook of Oral pathology, 6th edition.
5. Oral and maxillofacial pathology; Neville, Allen, 2nd edition.
6. Burket's Oral medicine diagnosis and treatment, 10th edition.
7. Principles of oral and maxillofacial surgery; U J Moore, 6th edition.
8. Medical problems in dentistry; Crispian Scully CBE, Roderick A Cawson, 5th edition.

Index